ADVANCE PRAISE FOR THE BIOMECHANICAL BRAIN

The Biomechanical Brain presents a rare, integrated perspective that respects neurological load, structural sequencing, and the realities of complex cases. From an upper cervical instability standpoint, the framework accurately reflects how overlooked cranio-cervical dysfunction can drive widespread symptoms—and why careful assessment and interdisciplinary thinking are essential. This is a thoughtful contribution for clinicians working beyond reductionist models.

— Dr. Sasha Blaskovich, DC
Director, Whiplash and Injury Clinic
Langley, BC, Canada – Bellingham, WA, USA

Brilliantly—at long last—The Biomechanical Brain places what has long been a difficult subject within the grasp of both inquisitive clinicians and patients. As an orthodontist, I can attest to the value of the collaborative therapeutic processes described in this book. The principles are explained in a clear, straightforward manner that makes complex interdisciplinary care understandable and applicable. Kudos to Geoff, and thank you.

— Dr. Duncan Brown, DDS
Envision Orthodontics
Canmore, AB, Canada

The Biomechanical Brain is a rare and essential work that dissolves the illusion of isolated function in the human body. It masterfully demonstrates that physiology is never an island—true understanding emerges only when bridges are built between structure, breath, bite, neurology, and adaptation. Through compelling clinical cases and thoughtful scientific integration, the authors reveal how fragmented thinking gives way to comprehensive clarity. The book offers not only insight, but a refined framework for risk management and intelligent treatment sequencing. It challenges silos, elevates collaboration, and empowers clinicians to see the whole before treating the part. A profound, paradigm-shifting contribution to modern healthcare.

— Dr. Christian Leonhardt, DDS, M.Sc.
Zahnärzte am Perlach
Augsburg, Germany

...From silos to systems. This book provides a timely and deeply insightful perspective on how the body truly functions as an integrated system. As a patient of the author and his colleagues/co-contributors, I can personally testify their interdisciplinary approach yields impactful life-changing results. As the CEO of two companies serving dentistry and orofacial health, I am excited to see how this book can empower interdisciplinary medicine and optimized patient care.

— Mark Maier
CEO, The Aurum Group; Co-CEO, FACE4D
Calgary, AB, Canada

The last time I checked, the rules of Biology and Physics don't care where you went to school or what degree you have." The tribalism of different professions, the different cultures of these professions, even natural preferences or biases all create a cloudy atmosphere of learning and consumption of information. The reality to all of this is that gems can be missed. The Biomechanical Brain takes on these realities and even doubles down by bringing together a dentist, a very uniquely specialized chiropractor, and a massage therapist. What won't be missed is a very unique perspective... in the effort to help learners do what they do – make other people's lives better.

— Dr Charlie Weingroff DPT ATC CSCS
West Palm Beach, FL – New York, NY – Los Angeles, CA, USA

THE BIOMECHANICAL BRAIN

REWIRING HEALTH FROM TEETH TO TOES

GEOFF DAKIN

WITH JEFF SCHOLTEN, DC
CURTIS WESTERSUND, DDS

The Biomechanical Brain
Rewiring Health from Teeth to Toes

First edition, 2026

Published by Vitruvian Publishing, Calgary, Alberta, Canada

Cover design by Rob Williams
Interior formatting by Hynek Palatin

To Dr. Jeff Scholten and Dr. Curtis Westersund—my colleagues, my teachers, and my partners in reimagining what modern healthcare can become.

For more than a decade, we have stood at the same table, each of us watching the same patient reveal a different truth. We came from three disciplines, three traditions, three vantage points, and somehow found our way to a shared language.

You challenged my assumptions and stretched my thinking. You helped me see what I had been missing, and reminded me—again and again—that no single profession ever owns the whole story.

This book was born in the space between us: in conversations that began as puzzles, in cases that refused to stay in their lanes, and in those rare moments of awe when a patient changed—not because someone worked harder, but because all three of us were finally looking in the same direction.

You are the reason this work became a framework rather than a collection of clinical wins. You are the reason this book exists.

With gratitude, respect, and enormous pride,
I dedicate this work to both of you.

Contents

Foreword

CONNECTING THE SILOS

TMD—often mistakenly called TMJ—is one of the most misunderstood pain conditions in modern healthcare. The confusion isn't limited to the public; it extends through dentistry, medicine, and nearly every profession that touches the patient in pain.

Every healthcare discipline exists for a valid reason. Each treats a specific part of the body, and each has become highly refined. But in the pursuit of specialization, we lost sight of the body as a whole. We began working in silos.

The dentist focuses on the bite. The chiropractor focuses on the spine. The massage therapist focuses on the muscles. The medical doctor focuses on symptoms and disease. Each sees only a fragment of the puzzle—yet the patient in pain does not live in fragments.

The pelvis, the spine—especially the upper cervical vertebrae—the jaw, and the bite are integral parts of one connected system. When one element falls out of alignment, the others compensate. When that compensation becomes overload, pain begins.

This book represents the work of three healthcare providers who refuse to remain in those silos: a neuromuscular dentist, a NUCCA chiropractor, and a massage therapist. We arrived from different directions, but reached the same conclusion: you cannot solve complex chronic pain by treating only one part of the body.

My fifty years as a dentist have left me in awe of the human body—its miraculous strengths and its frustrating weaknesses.

As I read this manuscript, I could immediately visualize the hips as the foundation of a building. A foundation that is twisted or torqued sets the stage for structural failure years down the line. Reading further, I recognized the spine's critical role in that foundation. The names of the first two vertebrae—Atlas and Axis—tell an important story. One holds the world; the other lets it spin. If they are not in harmony, distress travels both up and down the chain.

When considering how the bite connects to this system, I visualize a truss: a triangle formed by the two joints and the bite itself, helping stabilize the neck and the hips. If a condyle is jammed backward, the bite shifts and the triangle becomes crooked. Forces are no longer distributed evenly, and the muscles respond by bracing. Like a twisted truss in a building, the load has to go somewhere—and eventually, something starts to fail.

Real healing begins when the hip expert, the neck expert, and the bite expert work together—breaking down the silos. When alignment is restored from the ground up, and a balanced bite reinforces a balanced body rather than fighting it, many pain patterns resolve that once seemed mysterious, including the so-called "untreatable" condition known as TMD.

This book is written for the patient who has been passed from office to office with no clear answers. It is also for the practitioners who have quietly sensed there must be a better way, but were trained to stay in their lane.

When silos soften, when respect replaces rivalry, and when different hands work toward the same goal, the person in pain is no longer caught in the middle. They finally become the center of care again.

That is the purpose of this book.

Dr. Mac Lee, DDS, FAGD, FICCMO
Author of *The TMJ Trifecta: Solving Your Pain Puzzle* and *The Life Robbing Pain of TMD*

Introduction

WHY THIS BOOK EXISTS

For most people, pain begins as a question mark.

It might arrive quietly—a neck that never quite releases, a low back that flares without warning, a jaw that clicks or clenches for no obvious reason. Sometimes it follows trauma and has a clear beginning. More often it slips in sideways: tolerated at first, then accommodated, then defended against. Along the way, people are handed explanations that sound complete in isolation: muscular, mechanical, inflammatory, degenerative, stress-related, age-related, or simply "one of those things."

And then the search begins.

They find good practitioners—often excellent ones. A dentist improves the bite. A chiropractor restores motion. A physiotherapist strengthens what appears weak. A massage therapist reduces tone and tenderness. A breathing coach improves airflow. For a while, things feel better—sometimes dramatically so.

Then the symptoms return. Or migrate. Or reappear under a different name.

This book was born in that gap: the space between meaningful local improvement and the frustrating inability to make it last.

Over more than three decades in clinical practice, and through close collaboration with dentists, upper cervical chiropractors, and movement specialists, a pattern began to reveal itself—not as a theory, but as repeated clinical experience. The cases that failed were rarely poorly treated. They were incompletely framed. The body was being addressed in parts while behaving, predictably, as an integrated system.

Some of the most instructive lessons came not from failure, but from rare, unmistakable success: the patient whose chronic pain resolved when a distant piece of the puzzle was finally addressed; the case where world-class care had already been delivered, just not in the right order, or without the right integration. These weren't miracles. They were moments when the nervous system—relieved of an unrecognized burden—finally stopped spending its days fighting gravity.

What became clear across dancers and desk workers, dentists and chiropractors, elite athletes and chronically frustrated patients, was that these cases were not rare, mysterious, or especially complicated. They were predictable.

When pain persisted despite thoughtful, high-quality care; when symptoms shifted locations or returned without clear tissue injury; when posture, bite, breath, or balance improved briefly but refused to hold; when one practitioner succeeded locally only for the problem to reappear elsewhere—the pattern was remarkably consistent. The body wasn't necessarily failing at the site of pain. It was losing its ability to organize itself as a whole.

That is where single-discipline solutions quietly reach their limits—not because they are wrong, but because they are incomplete.

The Teeth-to-Toes collaboration emerged as a practical response to that recurring failure mode. Not a philosophy. Not a trend. An acknowledgment of something the body has been demonstrating all along: the pelvis, spine, airway, jaw, and nervous system are not separate problems to be handed off in sequence. They are interdependent parts of a single adaptive system—one that is constantly negotiating orientation, stability, and threat.

This book is for clinicians and patients who have sensed that truth firsthand, even when they lacked the language—or the framework—to name it.

What follows is not an argument for a new method, nor a turf war disguised as a hierarchy of who matters most. It is an exploration of how the body actually negotiates gravity, balance, and safety—and what happens when that negotiation quietly breaks down. To understand why teeth can influence toes, why a pelvis can distort breath, or why the nervous system clings to protective patterns long after danger has passed, we have to start where the body starts: not where pain announces itself, but where "upright" is decided.

That journey begins with orientation—where stability is negotiated, where the nervous system sets its reference points, and where the body learns how to hold itself in the world.

Welcome to *The Biomechanical Brain*.

A Note to Clinicians

HOW TO READ THIS BOOK

This book does not present a universal protocol, a fixed hierarchy of structures, or a single correct order of intervention. It offers a framework for clinical reasoning—not a recipe for treatment.

Primary Driver refers to the structure or issue currently placing the greatest load on the nervous system. It is not necessarily the site of pain, the most dramatic finding, or the structure emphasized by any single discipline. In different patients—and even in the same patient over time—what is primary can shift as load changes and compensation unwinds.

The chapters that follow are meant to be read relationally, not dogmatically. They illustrate how the nervous system reveals priority through assessment, response, and reassessment rather than dictating how care should be imposed based on theory alone.

To apply this model as a fixed sequence, to assume that one structure is always primary, or to bypass individual testing in favor of pattern recognition is to miss the point. The body is dynamic, and rigidity often undermines the very principles this work is built upon.

Effective care requires humility, ongoing assessment, and collaboration. The clinician's responsibility is not to enforce a sequence, but to discover it—and to respect the nervous system's capacity, timing, and tolerance for change.

PART ONE

Why You're Stuck

PROTECTION, LOAD, AND COMPENSATION

Before pain becomes a diagnosis, it is a strategy.

Before dysfunction becomes visible, it is protective.

This section explores how the nervous system manages load, how capacity quietly erodes, and how adaptation gradually becomes compensation. Understanding this progression is essential. Without it, treatment becomes guesswork. With it, patterns begin to make sense.

CHAPTER 1

The Body That Protects You

WHY PAIN IS A PROTECTIVE STRATEGY

Before pain becomes personal—before the hip locks, the neck tightens, or the back stiffens in a way that steals your breath—something quieter often begins unfolding inside the body.

Not an injury. Not a failure. Not degeneration.

Protection.

The human body is not built to chase pain; it is built to preserve stability, and pain is often what appears when that stability can no longer be protected quietly. Every day of your life, your nervous system works behind the scenes to keep you upright, balanced, and functional. It tracks gravity constantly. It monitors breath volume, visual input, joint position, muscle tone, emotional threat, airway resistance, and thousands of micro-signals you will never consciously feel.

It is one of the most sophisticated risk-management systems in biology.

And here is the part that reframes almost everything we think we know about chronic pain: the body protects you long before you ever notice it is doing so—and often long after it could afford to stop.

Pain is rarely the beginning. Pain is often the moment the body can no longer protect you quietly.

This book begins where pain truly begins: with the protective strategies the nervous system adopts when it can no longer trust its reference points—when it is forced to negotiate gravity without reliable orientation.

To understand this fully, we have to look past diagnoses and symptoms toward patterns: recurring strategies the nervous system uses to keep the head upright, the eyes level, and the system moving forward, whether or not the tissues below are happy about it.

If your training has been mostly mechanical—"the knee connects to the hip, the hip connects to the spine"—you're not wrong. You're just missing the conductor.

Bones and joints are the instruments. The nervous system is the one keeping time. And when the rhythm is threatened—when balance, breathing, or stability feels uncertain—the nervous system does what every intelligent system does: it chooses the strategy that preserves function today, even if that strategy comes with a cost tomorrow.

That cost is the hidden theme of chronic pain.

THE MISSING STEP: PREDICTION

There is a quiet step between stability and protection that's easy to miss unless you know to look for it: before the nervous system increases protection, it first predicts whether the body can remain stable. Every movement you make—standing up, reaching forward, turning your head—begins with the brain running a quick internal forecast about whether the system can manage the forces that are about to act upon it. That forecast is built from an astonishing volume of sensory information arriving every moment: joint position feedback, baseline muscle tone, vestibular input from the inner ear, visual orientation, breathing pressure, and even sensory signals from the jaw and neck. Out of all that data, the nervous system forms a prediction—can this body move safely under the demand that's coming next?

When the answer appears to be yes, movement tends to feel smooth and efficient, like the system is quietly confident. When the answer is uncertain, protection increases—not as a personality trait, not as a defect, but as a strategy. Muscle tone rises, movement becomes cautious, breathing patterns shift, posture adapts, and if the system stays in that state long enough, pain may eventually appear.

You can feel this process instantly in everyday life. Step onto solid pavement and you walk normally without thinking about it, but step onto ice and everything changes in a split second: your nervous system predicts instability and immediately modifies your movement—your muscles tighten, your steps shorten, and your whole body becomes careful. The nervous system doesn't wait for you to fall; it predicts instability and increases protection before anything goes wrong.

Seen this way, the body is constantly moving through a simple sequence:

Stability → Prediction → Protection

The nervous system evaluates stability, predicts whether it can safely manage the next demand, and increases protection when that prediction becomes uncertain. Once you begin seeing the body through this lens, many clinical puzzles start to make sense, because symptoms are rarely random—they are often the nervous system responding to a prediction about stability.

RACHEL: THE DANCER IN THE WHEELCHAIR

Rachel was sixteen. A dancer—the kind of mover whose disciplined presence made every room feel like an extension of a studio.

When she arrived at my clinic, she came in a wheelchair.

Her hip had seized so suddenly and so violently that she could no longer bear weight. Testing had been fruitless. Therapies had been even worse. Plenty of suspicions. No answers.

But the moment she stood for her assessment—balancing against the treatment table, breathing through tears—the real story surfaced.

Her pelvis wasn't merely rotated. It was spiraling. One side pushed forward while the other pulled backward, dramatically and unmistakably. Her rib cage twisted to counterbalance. Her diaphragm braced to contain the distortion. Her spine shaped itself to keep her upright and her eyes level. Her hip musculature clamped down in a last-ditch attempt to hold geometry that simply could not be held.

Her hip wasn't the problem. Her hip was the messenger.

Rachel didn't need someone to "fix her hip." She needed someone to understand what her hip had been protecting her from.

When her pelvis straightened, the change was breathtaking. Her breathing slowed. Her face softened. Her pain released.

I never saw that wheelchair again.

Within weeks she walked normally. Months later she was pain-free. Years later she was stronger than she had been since childhood.

But there's another key element to Rachel's case—and it's the unsettling one: she had been in that wheelchair for seven months while seeing skilled, respected clinicians, yet her pelvis had never been meaningfully assessed. Not because they weren't competent, but because the operating model they were using didn't force the question.

Her primary driver was hiding in plain sight.

That blind spot is exactly why this book exists.

Rachel's case teaches a foundational lesson that matters to every clinician who works with complex presentations: where pain shows up is often where protection has reached its limit, not where the story began.

We will return to Rachel later, because her story becomes even more instructive once you understand how primary drivers hide in plain sight—and why the order of correction determines whether a result holds.

For now, notice the central feature of the case: her system didn't fail. It protected brilliantly... until it couldn't.

KEN: THE OLYMPIAN WITH NO FOUNDATION

Ken was the opposite of fragile. An Olympic-level bobsleigh brakeman —explosive, powerful, built for force and velocity.

And yet his knees kept failing him: ACL tears, meniscal damage, a sports hernia, chronic pain, endless rehabilitation.

Everyone treated the knees. Of course they did. That's where the symptoms pointed.

But standing in front of me, the truth was just as unmistakable as it had been with Rachel.

His pelvis was severely distorted. Not a sport-specific asymmetry. Not a tidy adaptation to power production.

A structural liability.

Every stride, every lift, every acceleration out of the start gate—everything was being routed through a foundation that could not carry load cleanly. And when a foundation can't distribute force well, the nervous system does what it always does: it protects the next structure in line with bracing, altered timing, and compensatory stiffness.

Ken's system wasn't weak. It was managing risk.

When we corrected his pelvic alignment, the change was immediate. His gait reorganized. His knees tracked differently—perhaps for the first time in his life.

He completed his first pain-free competitive season in years.

Ken's story teaches the second foundational lesson: strength can compensate for distorted geometry—until the energy cost becomes unsustainable.

Performance can hide dysfunction for a long time. Elite capacity can delay symptoms. But it cannot rewrite physics.

We will return to Ken later as well, because his case illustrates a recurring blind spot in high-performance care: we often treat the stressed structure while missing the structure quietly distorting the entire force transfer strategy.

For now, hold the main point. His system protected his knees the best way it could—until protection became its own problem.

HOPE: THE NURSE AND THE UPRIGHT HEAD

Hope came in with chronic headaches—her primary complaint—but beneath them lived the same silent geometry I had seen in Rachel and Ken.

She was competent, caring, busy. Not dramatic. Not fragile. And she would not have described herself as someone with "a posture problem" until a fear began creeping in that she might be "folding forward," developing the beginning of a hunchback.

Her body wasn't failing cosmetically. It was coping neurologically.

Her pelvis was twisted. Her neck was overloaded simply trying to keep her head level. Her jaw was splinting—bracing, stabilizing—all day, every day. Her breathing was shallow not because she was anxious, but because the rib cage and diaphragm were living in a protective pattern.

Once her structure straightened and stabilized, her headaches receded for the first time in years. More importantly, she stopped living in a constant, low-grade fight with gravity.

Hope's case adds a crucial dimension: protection does not always announce itself as pain at the site of distortion. Often it appears upstream or downstream, disguised as headaches, jaw tension, dizziness, fatigue, or "mysterious" symptoms no scan can fully explain.

That is not psychosomatic. That is systems biology: a nervous system reallocating resources to keep you upright, oriented, and functional.

We will return to Hope later when we examine the upper gateways, because cases like hers make it almost impossible to understand chronic pain if you only think in local anatomy.

THE THREAD THAT BINDS THEM

Rachel. Ken. Hope. Different ages. Different lives. Different symptoms.

But one principle links them all: by the time symptoms appear, the nervous system has often been compensating for months—or years—trying to stabilize distortions you never felt happening.

Look closely at what their nervous systems were doing.

Rachel's system predicted instability and protected her hip.

Ken's system predicted instability and protected his knees.

Hope's system predicted instability and protected her neck and jaw.

Different structures. Different lives. The same underlying logic.

The nervous system sensed that stability could not be trusted, predicted that the system might not safely manage the loads passing through it, and increased protection in the region most capable of absorbing that risk.

Once you begin to see this pattern, the body stops looking mysterious. Symptoms stop looking random. They start looking like the nervous system doing exactly what it evolved to do—protect the organism when its prediction about stability becomes uncertain.

This is where modern care can get pulled off course, not because clinicians aren't skilled, but because pain is persuasive. It points. It demands attention. It creates a gravitational pull toward the loudest tissue in the room. Yet in case after case, the painful structure is not the starting point. It is the place where protection has finally reached its limit.

Karel Lewit, one of the great teachers of the Prague School, used to warn his students with blunt simplicity: "He who treats the site of pain is lost." Not because the painful area doesn't matter, but because it often isn't the driver. Treating it in isolation can become an endless loop: temporary relief, quiet recurrence, deeper compensation.

This reorganization is not random. It follows rules.

When the nervous system trusts its reference points, it runs movement like a well-tuned orchestra: efficient timing, shared load, quiet confidence. When it doesn't trust those reference points, it shifts into a different mode—bracing, gripping, breath holding, altered gait, altered tone. The goal is not elegance. The goal is survival with function.

That's why the "knee bone connected to the hip bone" model eventually breaks down in chronic pain. It's not that the anatomy is wrong. It's that anatomy alone doesn't explain why the system chose this strategy, why it's holding it, and why it resists change even when tissues look "fine."

The body doesn't just move. It negotiates. And negotiation has a cost.

That cost accumulates. Some bodies absorb it for a long time. Some can't. Some begin life with less reserve than we assume. Some acquire load silently through airway compromise, sleep fragmentation, old injuries, unresolved stress physiology, or years of compensating around asymmetry.

Eventually, the system reaches a threshold where protection can no longer remain quiet.

That's when symptoms "start." But clinically, symptoms are often the overflow, not the origin.

BRIDGE TO CHAPTER TWO

Before we talk about gateways—before we talk about pelvis, breath, bite, or the cranio-cervical junction—we need a model that explains something every clinician has seen but few can name cleanly:

Why two people can carry the same load and respond completely differently. Why one person bends and reorganizes while another breaks and spirals. Why one patient "should be better by now" but isn't. Why tissues can heal and symptoms can persist.

To answer that, we need to talk about capacity. We need to talk about the container the nervous system uses to measure threat.

We need to talk about the Threat Bucket.

That is where we go next.

CHAPTER 2

The Threat Bucket

WHY SOME SYSTEMS BEND AND OTHERS BREAK

Before pain appears—before muscles seize, breath rises, dizziness, fatigue, or anxiety enter the room—something quieter has often been happening inside the body.

Load accumulates.

In clinical practice we often talk about load as if it's mostly mechanical: tissue stress, strain, compression, shear. That's part of the story. But it's not the whole story in complex, persistent cases.

The nervous system experiences load more like a bucket experiences water: a drop at a time.

A stressor here. A shift there. A night of poor sleep. A week of elevated sympathetic tone. A month of shallow breathing. A year of compensating around asymmetry. A decade of fighting to maintain a compromised airway. Add illness, hormonal shifts, inflammatory noise, and the low-grade vigilance that becomes someone's baseline without them ever naming it as "stress."

Most people feel none of this in real time. But the nervous system tracks it. It adapts—brilliantly—until it can't. And when it can no longer protect quietly, it spills.

What is actually changing inside the nervous system during this accumulation is its prediction about stability.

As the bucket fills, the brain becomes less confident that the body can safely manage the forces acting upon it. The tissues may not have failed. The joints may not be damaged. But the nervous system begins to sense that the system is operating closer to its limits.

When that prediction shifts, protection increases.

Muscles tighten in places that were previously quiet. Breathing patterns change. Movement becomes cautious. Postural strategies appear that redistribute load in ways the person may never consciously notice.

Nothing in the body is malfunctioning in this moment. The nervous system is doing exactly what it evolved to do: adjusting its level of protection based on its prediction about stability.

Seen this way, the Threat Bucket is not just a container for stress. It is the context that shapes the nervous system's expectations about what the body can safely handle.

When the bucket is relatively empty, the system predicts safety and movement flows easily.

When the bucket approaches its limit, the system predicts risk—and protection increases accordingly.

Not as weakness. Not as failure.

As symptoms.

Pain. Headaches. Dizziness. Muscle guarding. Digestive disruption. Fatigue. Jaw tension. Rib stiffness. Strange sensations no scan can explain. Sudden instability. Or the unnerving sense that the body is "slipping out of place."

Patients can spend years treating the overflow without ever being taught to look for the bucket.

This chapter is the bucket—because the bucket is capacity, the bucket is history, and the bucket is biology. In many chronic pain patients, it also matters to say plainly: the bucket did not start empty.

THE CLINICAL PURPOSE OF THE THREAT BUCKET MODEL

The Threat Bucket is not a poetic metaphor. It is a practical way to organize what you already know:

Why identical tissue findings can produce different symptom burdens.

Why the "same" accident can produce wildly different recovery trajectories.

Why symptoms can persist long after expected tissue-healing windows.

Why some interventions create brief relief, then rebound.

Why a patient can appear calm, motivated, and compliant—and still remain physiologically defended.

If a clinician tries to solve complex cases with a purely local model—"treat the painful structure"—they will eventually meet the ceiling of that approach. The Threat Bucket is one of the simplest ways to step beyond that ceiling without drifting into vague psychology or ideology.

The bucket has two governing variables:

How fast it fills (total input load).

How well it drains (restoration, recovery, regulation, and clarity).

Most chronic pain patients don't have a "mystery condition." They have a system where filling has outpaced draining for too long.

HOW BUCKETS FILL

Load is rarely one thing. It's the sum of many small forces acting at once, often in silence:

Mechanical load: asymmetry, joint compression, altered gait, bracing patterns, repetitive strain.

Respiratory load: a rib cage that doesn't expand well, a diaphragm that behaves like a brace, chronic mouth breathing.

Sensory-motor load: distorted proprioception, vestibular mismatch, visual dependence, protective reflexes firing too often.

Autonomic load: persistent sympathetic tone, poor vagal recovery, fragmented sleep.

Metabolic/inflammatory load: blood sugar volatility, nutrient depletion, illness, persistent background noise.

Cognitive-emotional load: vigilance, perfectionism, unresolved trauma, chronic uncertainty—even when the person would never label it "stress."

None of these categories is controversial. What is often missed is what happens when several are present at once: the system begins to protect everywhere to stabilize anything.

In that state, pain is not always a sign of tissue damage. Pain is often the nervous system's signal that the cost of protection has become too high.

WHY THE BUCKET SPILLS

Symptoms are overflow, not origin.

The spill point is the moment the nervous system can no longer maintain a protective strategy quietly. Clinically, that changes how we interpret "new" symptoms. A flare-up is not always a new injury. It is often a system reaching threshold.

That's why "nothing showed up on imaging" is such a common feature of these cases. Many of the most disabling chronic patterns are not a failure of structure to hold together; they are a failure of capacity to keep paying the energetic cost of compensation.

In complex cases, the decisive question becomes less philosophical and more strategic:

What is filling the bucket—and what is preventing it from draining?

MARYANNE: WHEN A SYSTEM WITH LITTLE RESERVE RUNS OUT

Maryanne moved through life with the careful grace of someone carrying something fragile. Soft-spoken. Steady. Impeccably composed in the way people become when discomfort is constant but responsibilities do not wait.

She travelled from Toronto to Calgary to begin care—an act of resolve in itself—but had barely started when she discovered she was pregnant. Rehab was paused. Pregnancy, like all pregnancies, reshaped her body in expected ways and in ways she didn't fully understand.

The truth was simple: her bucket was already half full before life began adding more.

Her connective tissue told the story early: hypermobile, elastic, effortless to demonstrate. Less effortless to live inside.

Hypermobility is not a character flaw, and it isn't simply "being flexible." It often reflects connective tissue that behaves differently—less passive restraint, more give than most—so the nervous system has to generate stability actively, all day, every day. That can be an advantage in dance, gymnastics, and contortion. It can also be a double-edged sword in ordinary life, because the cost of keeping joints organized is higher and the margin for recovery is smaller.

Her pelvis had been drifting for years. Her diaphragm behaved more like a splint than a pump. Breath lived high in her chest. Sleep was light. Stress was quiet but constant. Her neck and bite added their own complications to an already overloaded system.

By the time she returned postpartum, her symptoms were stacking: neck tightness, headaches, low-back discomfort, hip pulling, and the unnerving sense that her body was always on the verge of shifting out of place.

Nothing dramatic. Nothing a scan would dignify.

Everything adding load.

One morning she said something that captured the physiology better than any label: "I wake up tired, like I spent the whole night trying to hold myself together."

That is the language of a full bucket.

When we reduced one of the largest contributors to her internal load —by straightening pelvic mechanics—her system softened quickly. Not because one correction fixed everything, but because the nervous system finally received evidence that the cost of stabilization had dropped.

Her breath slowed and deepened. Sleep improved. Headaches eased. The daily sensation of vigilance in her own body quieted.

Maryanne wasn't delicate. She was overloaded.

And overloaded systems don't fail because they're weak. They struggle because they've been asked to defend too much for too long.

CLARITY, CONFUSION, AND THREAT

One of the most underestimated contributors to load is uncertainty.

We often talk about pain as if it's driven by "damage" or by "sensitivity." In many chronic cases, the more useful lever is neither of those.

It's clarity.

The nervous system depends on continuous streams of information—proprioception, vestibular input, vision, and interoception—to predict what is happening and what is about to happen. When those signals are coherent, the system runs efficiently. When they are distorted or contradictory, the system protects.

This is one reason well-intentioned interventions can fail. Effort does not automatically create safety. Intensity does not automatically create clarity. "Feeling more" is not the same as "moving better."

When the brain can't accurately map movement, timing, or load distribution, it often fills the gaps with protection: bracing, gripping, breath holding, jaw clenching, and movement avoidance.

These are not personality traits. They are strategies. And strategies have an energy cost.

Confusion is threat. Clarity is relief. Relief is what allows the bucket to begin draining.

WHEN SURVIVAL OVERRIDES REST

When threat accumulates faster than the system can adapt, the body shifts into chronic defense. This is where autonomic physiology becomes clinically relevant, not as abstraction but as lived experience.

Sleep fragments. Digestion slows. Breath becomes shallow. Muscles brace compulsively. The limbic system becomes watchful, then hyper-watchful.

A person may describe this as "tension," "anxiety," or "fatigue." Or they may describe nothing at all beyond pain and stiffness. The body does not need the patient to be psychologically distressed to behave physiologically threatened.

This is not weakness. It is a system prioritizing survival over restoration.

And the reason this matters is strategic: a nervous system in chronic defense often resists change—especially sudden change—even when the change is beneficial. That resistance is often misread as noncompliance, catastrophizing, or "failure to engage." More often, it is protection from a system with no reserve.

The hopeful part is equally physiological. When mechanical load decreases, breathing improves, and clarity returns, autonomic tone can shift. When autonomic tone shifts, sleep improves. When sleep improves, recovery becomes possible. And when recovery becomes possible, the bucket finally drains.

HYPERMOBILITY: WHEN PASSIVE STABILITY IS LOW, THE SYSTEM GETS LOUD

In some bodies, connective tissue provides less passive restraint. The "hardware" is simply more elastic than average—often wonderful for dancers, gymnasts, and contortionists, and often exhausting for everyone else. When passive restraint is low, the nervous system has to generate more active stability to feel safe.

That extra stability doesn't usually arrive as calm strength. It often arrives as vigilance: bracing, gripping, scanning, clenching, micromanaging posture, reacting strongly to small changes.

This is not a personality flaw. It is a strategy—the nervous system turning the volume up because the usual quiet feedback from joints and connective tissue is less reliable.

This matters because it reframes "difficult cases." In a hypermobile system, symptoms are often not just overflow; they're overflow plus instability. When instability and a full bucket coexist, the nervous system tends to defend harder, recover slower, and tolerate less aggressive change.

DEVELOPMENTAL LOAD: HISTORY LIVES IN THE BODY

Some buckets begin filling long before adulthood.

Childhood mouth breathing reshapes facial bones. A narrow palate crowds the bite. A restricted airway encourages forward-head orientation. Forward-head orientation increases demand at the cranio-cervical junction. Altered upper cervical mechanics distort proprioceptive input. Distorted proprioception increases protective tone.

It's a cascade. Not cosmetic. Neurological.

By adulthood, most people don't identify this as "an airway story." They simply report patterns clinicians recognize immediately once they know to look: shoulders living too close to ears, a neck that never feels off-duty, a jaw that behaves like a clamp, a rib cage that doesn't expand well posteriorly, and a breath that never seems to drop.

Breath often told the truth years before pain was given the microphone.

A STORY WE WILL RETURN TO

Some buckets overflow slowly, like Maryanne's. Some fill gradually but relentlessly. And some spill suddenly—the right event landing in a system already at its limit.

Kim's story begins with a motor-vehicle accident she appeared to "walk away from," until the hours that followed revealed the truth: jaw rigidity, dizziness, headaches, cognitive fog, neck stiffness, and a body that could no longer organize itself under load.

We will return to Kim later, because her case sits precisely at the intersection of the gateways and the clinical question of order.

For now, she belongs here for one reason: overflow is not a symptom. It is a state. And if we treat overflow like a local problem, we keep missing the operating system.

WHERE ALIGNMENT FITS INTO THE BUCKET

Alignment is not aesthetic. It's metabolic and neurological cost.

A twisted pelvis alters proprioception. A rotated rib cage changes breath mechanics. A diaphragm that cannot descend increases autonomic load. A forward head increases demand at the CCJ. A dysfunctional bite distorts cranial tension patterns.

None of this is cosmetic. All of it is threat.

When alignment improves, breath often slows and deepens. Tone softens. Coordination improves. Muscles stop behaving like splints. The nervous system reclaims capacity that used to be spent on protection.

The bucket doesn't merely stop filling. It begins to drain.

THE HEART OF TEETH-TO-TOES

Every discipline inside a Teeth-to-Toes model—dentistry, upper cervical care, corrective exercise, manual therapy, nutrition, breath restoration—should share one biological goal:

Reduce threat. Restore capacity. Drain the bucket.

As capacity returns, movement becomes fluid. Breathing becomes grounded. Flare-ups become shorter, rarer, easier to manage. Sleep becomes restorative. The nervous system stops interpreting ordinary life as an ongoing threat.

This is the beginning of resilience.

WHY THIS CHAPTER MATTERS

Conventional healthcare asks, "Where does it hurt?"

A systems-aware clinician asks, "What is filling the bucket—and what prevents it from draining?"

Symptoms mark the overflow. The bucket explains the pattern. Most importantly, this model protects both clinician and patient from a common failure mode: treating overflow forever while the bucket continues to fill.

Seen through this lens, the nervous system is not simply reacting to injury or stress—it is continuously predicting whether the body can remain stable under the demands placed upon it. As the bucket fills, those predictions become more cautious, and protection begins to appear in places that may seem unrelated to the original load. What looks like stiffness, pain, guarding, or fatigue is often the system responding to a simple question it is constantly asking: Can this body safely manage what comes next?

BRIDGE TO CHAPTER THREE

If Chapter One introduced protection as the operating logic of the system, this chapter gave you the container that explains why protection becomes chronic.

Now we take the next step—because buckets do not fill randomly. They fill through strategies.

And one strategy, more than any other, explains why chronic patterns become so stubborn: compensation that once helped becomes the thing that keeps the system trapped.

That is where we go next.

CHAPTER 3

When Adaptation Becomes Compensation

THE TURNING POINT IN EVERY PAIN STORY

If Chapter Two introduced the Threat Bucket—how load accumulates, how capacity varies, and why systems spill—this chapter names the moment the bucket stops being theoretical and becomes unmistakably clinical: the point where adaptation crosses a line and turns into compensation.

Before pain announces itself—before anything stiffens, spasms, burns, or "goes out"—the nervous system has usually been working quietly in the background for a long time. It has been negotiating gravity, stabilizing reference points, and redistributing force without asking for your permission or your attention. That process is adaptation. It isn't weakness. It's one of the most intelligent things the neuromuscular system does.

When capacity is high and threat is manageable, adaptation is nearly invisible. People don't feel it. They don't name it. They just live. But capacity is not infinite, and when life starts asking more than the system can sustainably give, adaptation becomes expensive. It stops being an elegant adjustment and becomes a protective strategy—one that consumes resources. That is compensation.

Where adaptation preserves coherence, compensation distorts it. Where adaptation manages load efficiently, compensation spends capacity aggressively. And once a system begins spending more than it can afford, the bucket doesn't just fill—it fills faster, because the very strategies used to cope add more load to the total. This is one reason chronic pain is so confusing to both patients and clinicians. It isn't that the body "breaks" suddenly. It's that the system runs out of affordable options, and the options that remain are protective.

What has changed in that moment is not just mechanics—it is the nervous system's prediction about stability.

Earlier in the book we introduced a simple sequence that governs how the body manages risk: stability → prediction → protection. As long as the nervous system predicts that stability can be maintained, adaptation remains efficient and largely invisible. Movement flows, load distributes cleanly, and the system quietly solves problems without demanding attention.

But when the prediction shifts—when the brain becomes less confident that the body can safely manage the forces moving through it—the strategy changes.

Protection increases.

Compensation is often the visible expression of that shift. The system borrows stability from somewhere else. One region stiffens so another can move. One joint becomes a brace so another can remain functional. The body spends capacity to preserve control.

Nothing about this is accidental. It is the nervous system solving a stability problem with the tools it still has available.

The difficulty is that compensation solves today's problem by borrowing from tomorrow's capacity. Over time the borrowed stability becomes expensive, and the bucket begins to fill faster than it drains.

CONNECTEDNESS: THE ONE LESSON WE ALL RECEIVED

Most clinicians were trained in parts: regions, specialties, discrete diagnoses, and local tissue narratives. Meanwhile, most patients were trained in only one body-wide concept—and they learned it as children: "The knee bone's connected to the hip bone..."

It's crude. It's catchy. It's also more clinically important than most people realize, because complex pain rarely belongs to one structure in isolation. It belongs to patterns: interlocking strategies that spread load, borrow stability from one region to protect another, and keep the system upright at a cost. This chapter is where that "Dem Bones" truth becomes useful, because the shift from adaptation to compensation is the moment those connections stop being academic and start becoming diagnostic.

WHY THIS MATTERS FOR EXERCISE

One reason compensation persists—sometimes for years—is that we keep prescribing demand to a system that is already defending. Exercise is often treated as inherently positive, as though movement is always restorative and "more" is automatically better. That worldview is understandable, even well-intentioned, but it routinely traps people who are conscientious, disciplined, and doing everything they believe is correct.

Exercise is not neutral input. Like any meaningful intervention, it places demand on the nervous system: coordination demand, load demand, timing demand, and tolerance demand. Some exercises reduce threat and restore capacity by improving clarity and decreasing protective tone. Others increase threat by amplifying load and complexity in a system that cannot currently afford them.

We intuitively accept that pharmaceutical prescriptions are individual, dose-dependent, and time-sensitive. Exercise prescriptions follow the same rules—yet they're often delivered as generic routines, an approach that works beautifully for robust systems and fails quietly for overloaded ones. When capacity is low and protection is high, even "good" exercises can become another stressor the system must defend against. The response pattern is predictable: more bracing, shallower breathing, jaw clenching, increased asymmetry, delayed recovery, and the sense that progress is always temporary.

In persistent pain, the goal is not to prove discipline or accumulate effort. The goal is to restore capacity. Until capacity returns, the nervous system will continue to prioritize safety over performance—no matter how appropriate the exercise looks on paper. This is not a failure of motivation. It is often a failure of timing.

And it leads to a pattern most clinicians have seen—even if they've never named it.

THE DAKIN EFFECT: WHEN "GOOD EXERCISE" BECOMES ASYMMETRIC LOAD

The Dakin Effect describes a clinical reality that contradicts a near-universal belief: that exercise is usually beneficial and, at worst, neutral. In an overloaded system, the same exercise can be helpful—or neutral—on one side and measurably destabilizing on the other.

You'll see it with something as standard as a Couch Stretch. Done on one side, a person may stand a little straighter, feel looser, or show no meaningful change. Done on the other side, the same stretch can drive the ilium outside a healthy range, recreate a functional leg-length difference, or worsen weightbearing symmetry. Nothing about the exercise is inherently "bad." The problem is the system receiving it.

For Teeth-to-Toes patients—those carrying a layered mix of lower-body malalignment, upper cervical disorganization, and bite-driven sensory noise—exercise is often neither beneficial nor neutral. It can be anti-therapeutic: it adds load, increases compensation, and teaches the nervous system a more expensive strategy. So the Dakin Effect is not a warning about effort. It's a warning about dose, side, and sequence.

Julie is the case that made that lesson unavoidable.

JULIE: THE BODY THAT RAN OUT OF OPTIONS

Julie's story did not begin with back pain. It did not begin with the jaw. It didn't even begin with the headaches that eventually stole whole days from her life. Her story began years earlier with a dental appliance—an intervention designed to help, but one her nervous system could not afford at that moment in her sequence.

She wore it faithfully, adjusted it, tried again and again. The result was not relief. Instead, she developed episodes of jaw locking—sudden periods where the jaw clamped shut for minutes or hours and then released without a clear explanation. This is the moment where many clinicians start debating labels, but the more useful interpretation was simpler: her system was signaling overload in the language it had available.

Her dentist eventually reached the edge of the map and referred her for upper cervical care. That intervention helped dramatically: headaches softened, neck tone reduced, and her overall reactivity decreased. It was a real win—just not a complete one—because her lower back remained unchanged. It was stubborn, protective, and unresponsive to everything that "should have helped."

When Julie arrived in my treatment room, the picture sharpened the moment she stood. Her pelvis was locked in a full torsion pattern—one side pulled forward, the other dragged backward. This wasn't a minor asymmetry. It was a structural conflict that forced every region above it to negotiate gravity at a premium.

Seen through that lens, her history stopped looking fragmented. Her jaw had not failed her. Her neck had not failed her. Her back had not failed her. They had been protecting her—each compensating in its own way—because the system below could not provide a reliable reference.

When we corrected her pelvic mechanics, her presentation changed quickly. Breath slowed and deepened. Global tone softened. Her back pain eased in a way she had not experienced for years. More importantly, something became visible that is often hidden until load drops: the order of the problem—not as ideology, not as a checklist, but as clinical logic.

When the system is overloaded, you rarely see the full map. You see whatever is loudest. As the bucket drains, the next limiter becomes detectable, and the clinician's job is to recognize that shift rather than forcing the same intervention harder. Julie asked a question she had not been able to ask for nearly a decade: was it time to revisit the dental component of her care? We will return to that question later, because it sits precisely at the intersection of gateways and sequencing. For now, Julie's story teaches a principle that governs everything that follows: you cannot accurately prescribe demand to a system that is still defending.

WHY UPPER CERVICAL HELPED, BUT COULD NOT FINISH

Upper cervical care addressed what could be assessed and stabilized at the time, and it mattered. But the foundation below was still driving the global pattern. A significantly torsioned pelvis can distort proprioception and force transfer so deeply that upstream findings often function as secondary adaptations rather than primary drivers. In that scenario, even excellent upper cervical or dental work may be partially expressed—then gradually pulled back into protection by what remains unresolved beneath it.

This is not a critique of any discipline. It's a statement about hierarchy. When compensation is entrenched, partial wins are common. They are not failures; they are signals that the system is reorganizing in layers. The clinician's job is to notice what the partial win reveals about the next step rather than concluding the intervention "didn't work."

Julie's history finally made sense: improvements that didn't hold, stubborn losses, and relief that faded. The interventions were not wrong. They were delivered into a system that still had to defend.

WHEN LOAD EXCEEDS CAPACITY

When threat outweighs capacity, the system shifts from efficiency to survival—and that shift has recognizable features. The diaphragm behaves like a brace, the rib cage stiffens to create stability, tongue posture collapses, the jaw clamps, gait becomes less symmetrical, proprioception fragments, and the autonomic nervous system trends toward sympathetic dominance. The patient experiences this not as a philosophical state, but as lived reality: heightened tone, reduced tolerance, increased reactivity, and the sense that the body is always negotiating rather than moving.

Protection is not pathology. It is strategy. But protection is expensive. Eventually, the budget runs out.

WHERE JULIE STANDS NOW

Julie is no longer drowning in compensation. Her pelvis is stabilizing. Her upper cervical system is settling. Her symptoms are reorganizing as the bucket drains. Only now can questions like bite involvement be evaluated with the precision they require. Not every patient needs dental work. Not every bite is a driver. Not every jaw imbalance requires hardware. But when bite mechanics do matter, it is often only visible once the system beneath has stopped screaming for protection.

Julie is standing at that threshold—the point where the next step becomes visible. Her story is no longer chaotic. It is coherent.

BRIDGE TO CHAPTER FOUR

Adaptation and compensation are not mistakes. They are the nervous system doing exactly what it was designed to do. But once compensation becomes the dominant strategy—once the system is spending more than it can afford—a different chapter begins. Symptoms multiply. Function degrades. Margin disappears. The patient experiences something that is both deeply physical and deeply confusing: the body begins to fight itself.

That is where we go next.

CHAPTER 4

When the Body Fights Itself

HOW COMPENSATION BECOMES OVERLOAD, AND OVERLOAD BECOMES SUFFERING

If Chapter Three named the turning point—when adaptation quietly becomes compensation—this chapter follows the next, more consequential shift: what happens when compensation stops being an occasional strategy and becomes the nervous system's default operating system.

By the time pain becomes intolerable—by the time symptoms feel "mysterious," unpredictable, or frightening—something important has often already changed inside the patient. The body is no longer adapting in the background while life continues in the foreground. The body is surviving.

Compensation is not the villain of this book. In the early stages, it can be brilliant: a temporary bridge that allows a person to stay functional, stay employed, keep parenting, keep training, keep showing up. But every bridge has a load limit. When a system remains in compensation too long—or when incoming load exceeds remaining capacity—the bridge becomes the bottleneck. The nervous system crosses into a new physiological state: overwhelm.

This is the moment the body begins fighting itself—not maliciously, but mechanically, neurologically, chemically, and reflexively. Past this threshold, the system spends more energy bracing than moving, defending than sensing, and surviving than restoring. That is the true beginning of chronic pain: not as a local tissue story, but as a whole-system state.

At this stage something subtle but decisive has shifted inside the nervous system: its prediction about safety. Earlier in the book we described how the brain constantly evaluates stability, predicts whether the body can manage the forces acting upon it, and increases protection when that prediction becomes uncertain. In a system living near overwhelm, those predictions become chronically cautious. Movements that once felt ordinary are now interpreted as potential threats. Small perturbations demand large responses. The nervous system begins operating with a narrower margin for error, raising baseline tone and maintaining defensive strategies long after the original mechanical challenge has passed. What the patient experiences as tension, fragility, or hypersensitivity is often the physiological expression of a brain that no longer expects the body to remain stable without constant protection.

THE TIPPING POINT: WHEN COMPENSATION LOSES ITS GRACE

In the beginning, compensation can look almost elegant. A subtle rib rotation improves airflow. A small jaw shift reduces cranial strain. A mild pelvic torsion buys mechanical advantage that keeps gait functional and pain intermittent. These are not "errors." They are strategies —often the best strategies available at the time.

But as threat accumulates and capacity shrinks, compensation becomes urgent. The signs are familiar to anyone who treats complex pain patients: movement stiffens, breath migrates upward, vision narrows, neck flexors overwork, hip stabilizers fatigue, and the diaphragm tightens into armor. The atlas strains relentlessly for midline while everything below it drifts. At that point, the body is attempting three jobs at once: hold alignment together—however imperfectly; generate enough bracing to prevent collapse; and still meet the demands of normal life. The system is not failing. It is spending more than it can afford.

Many clinicians assume the primary threats to alignment are dramatic injuries or rare anatomical anomalies. Those exist, and we should respect them. Some individuals carry congenital variations—an unusually shaped atlas, asymmetrical occipital condyles, or a bite that never centered—and those differences can matter. But they are not the common story in modern chronic pain.

The more universal story is quieter: the nervous system can generate asymmetry all by itself. All it requires is time, repetitive load, habit, and the friction of living inside a body that keeps protecting long after protection has become costly. Structural differences may sketch the blueprint. Functional asymmetry writes the story. Most imbalances are not congenital. They are learned, accumulated, practiced. They are the nervous system's best ideas—long after those ideas stop serving it.

Julie, from the previous chapter, arrived at that edge: a body that had run out of affordable strategies. But there is another category of patient —one where the system reaches overwhelm not gradually, but explosively. In those cases, the clinical challenge is not simply "fixing posture" or "building strength." The challenge is restoring tolerance, clarity, and stability to a system that has lost its reference points.

SEAN: WHEN THE NERVOUS SYSTEM SLIPS OUT OF NEUTRAL

Sean was a teenager when the trouble began. First came shoulder pain — strange and stubborn, appearing without a clear mechanical explanation. His mother sought care from massage therapists, chiropractors, and well-meaning specialists. Several interventions helped briefly, which is often what makes these cases so misleading: temporary improvement can make it feel like you're close—even when the system is deteriorating under the surface.

Then the symptoms multiplied: neck pain, back pain, headaches, nausea, sleep disruption, loss of appetite—a nervous system behaving as though danger were everywhere. By the time he arrived in my clinic, his presentation had the unmistakable quality of a system clinging to orientation by its fingernails.

His pelvis was distorted. His spine showed signs consistent with hypermobility. His head hovered forward as though searching for stability that was no longer reliably available. And his nervous system was loud: reactive, hyper-alert, easily startled—an organism interpreting subtle shifts as major threats. His Cervical Syndrome Test was clearly positive.

This was not simply a mechanical problem. It was neurological overwhelm wearing mechanical clothing.

I referred him immediately for upper cervical care. Imaging confirmed what the exam suggested: upper cervical misalignment, a stressed cranio-cervical junction, and instability patterns that no amount of strengthening, stretching, or soft-tissue work could resolve in isolation.

Over the following years—not weeks—Sean moved through a carefully paced, multidisciplinary plan: upper cervical correction and monitoring; specialized cervical evaluation; manual therapy and nonaggressive corrective exercise; lifestyle changes to reduce autonomic load; and progression slow enough that his nervous system could tolerate change without rebounding into protection.

I have rarely seen a clearer example of a nervous system that had slipped fully out of neutral—and then, slowly and methodically, found its way back. Today, his life resembles the life of a young man again. But the path was long, delicate, and profoundly instructive.

Sean's case teaches a truth clinicians ignore at their peril: when the nervous system is overwhelmed, no structure—not even a corrected one—can reliably hold its improvements. Stability is not only a matter of alignment. It is a matter of capacity.

We will return to Sean later, because his case becomes even more illuminating once the Four Gateways are on the table and sequencing becomes explicit. For now, he serves as our clearest example of what overwhelm looks like when it becomes systemic.

THE MECHANICS OF OVERWHELM

When adaptive bandwidth is exceeded, three processes often begin unfolding at the same time—each feeding the other.

First, alignment destabilizes. Pelvic torsion increases. The rib cage stiffens and rotates to create artificial stability. The diaphragm braces. The atlas strains for midline. The jaw clamps to splint the system. The airway can narrow and breathing becomes shallow, high, and defensive. The patient experiences this as tightness, fragility, and "never quite finding neutral."

Second, sensory processing degrades. Proprioception fragments. Balance becomes unreliable. Muscle sequencing deteriorates. Joint position becomes harder to perceive. The clinician sees it as inconsistent motor control, rapid fatigue, and a system that can't integrate cues —even good ones—without increasing protection.

Third, autonomic tone shifts toward survival. Heart rate variability drops. Sympathetic tone stays elevated. Sleep loses its restorative quality. The limbic system amplifies threat detection. The patient becomes more reactive, more sensitive, and less resilient—not because they are weak-minded, but because their physiology is flooded.

In other words, the body loses mechanical clarity and neurological clarity at the same time. This—not tissue damage—is the defining feature of chronic pain as a state.

THE CCJ AND THE BITE: TWO POWERFUL AMPLIFIERS

Once compensation becomes global, two regions often absorb disproportionate burden because they sit at critical neurological choke points.

The cranio-cervical junction (CCJ) is one. The atlas must maintain head orientation even as everything below it drifts. At first it adapts. Then it stabilizes. Then it strains. Eventually, it can lose the ability to locate neutral reliably. This is where headaches can emerge, neck fatigue becomes constant, visual strain accumulates, and dizziness can enter the picture. Importantly, many of these symptoms don't behave like simple "neck pain," because the CCJ isn't merely musculoskeletal—it's a sensory hub with survival implications when orientation becomes unreliable.

The bite is the other. When the body cannot stabilize from below, the jaw attempts to stabilize from above. The bite becomes a steering mechanism. The jaw becomes a splint. The teeth become part of the postural system. Clenching becomes habitual. Grinding intensifies. Masseter and temporalis tone becomes reflexive and resistant to release.

Neither region was designed to carry foundational load. But they will —if they must. And when they do, the nervous system pays dearly.

WHEN HEALING ACTUALLY BEGINS

Julie showed us the moment compensation hits its limit. Sean showed us what it looks like when overwhelm becomes systemic. Together, they point to a truth that reframes recovery for both clinicians and patients: the body does not fundamentally heal when pain decreases. It often begins healing when load decreases and capacity returns.

This is why symptom management can produce partial wins while the underlying state remains unchanged. A patient may feel better for a day, a week, even a month—and still be living in a system that cannot tolerate normal life without rebuilding protection. The turning point is not the perfect exercise, the perfect adjustment, or the perfect orthotic. It is the moment the nervous system recognizes—through improved clarity and reduced demand—I have enough capacity to reorganize again.

That recognition is not philosophical. It is physiological. It is visible in breathing, gait, sleep, tone, and recovery time, and it is often felt by the patient as something surprisingly simple: space.

BRIDGE TO CHAPTER FIVE

If this chapter described what happens when compensation becomes overwhelm, the next chapter asks the question that determines outcomes: why do some bodies survive overload by becoming stronger — while others survive by becoming more protective?

This is where the rehab world gets fooled. Some compensation patterns create performance. Others create suffering. Often, they look similar at first glance. The difference is not the athlete's character, or the patient's willpower, or the therapist's technique. The difference is the relationship between load and capacity—and the cost of the strategy being used to survive.

In Chapter Five we step into The Athlete's Paradox, where adaptation can become advantage, compensation can become liability, and the line between them decides everything.

That is where we go next.

CHAPTER 5

The Athlete's Paradox

WHY THE STRONGEST BODIES BREAK THE HARDEST

If Chapter Four described what it looks like when a system crosses into overwhelm—when compensation becomes the dominant state—this chapter clarifies why high performers can live in that state longer than anyone expects, and why the eventual consequences can be so dramatic.

In sport, we are trained to respect outputs: speed, strength, skill, tolerance, work ethic. The athlete is the person who can keep producing while everyone else is forced to stop, which is precisely why athletic bodies often fool clinicians. They do not present like fragile systems. They present like resilient ones.

But performance is not the same as capacity.

Capacity is the quiet bandwidth beneath the surface—the margin the nervous system relies on to manage threat, organize alignment, coordinate breath mechanics, distribute load, and absorb the normal friction of life. When that bandwidth is plentiful, the athlete looks durable because they are durable. When that bandwidth shrinks, the athlete can still look durable—right up until they can't.

This is the athlete's paradox: the most capable bodies are often the ones that can compensate so effectively that they delay obvious warning signs. They keep playing. They keep training. They keep "working through it." The system remains functional not because it is problem-free, but because it is resourceful. For clinicians, that distinction matters. It changes what we look for and how we interpret early symptoms.

In the general population, early signs of trouble are often loud and local: a low back that seizes, a knee that swells, a shoulder that loses range. In elite performers, the early signs can be subtle and easily dismissed: asymmetrical fatigue, a stride that feels "off," a minor loss of efficiency, a recovery curve that is just a little slower than it should be. In other words, athletes often report performance changes long before they report pain, and when pain finally arrives, it may not arrive gradually. Average bodies tend to buckle early. Athletic bodies tend to buckle late. Late, however, does not mean gently. It often means abruptly—because the buffer that was hiding the distortion has already been spent.

To be clear, this is not an argument against sport-specific asymmetry. Many elite performances are built on side dominance and rotational bias, and that kind of asymmetry can be advantageous; it may even be necessary for world-class output. The concern here is non-advantageous distortion: patterns that raise the cost of doing business without improving output. No athlete benefits from tibial torsion, genu valgum, pelvic torsion, CCJ malalignment, or a TMJ system recruited as a stabilizer. Those are not performance adaptations. Those are load.

So the question becomes clinical, not philosophical: is the athlete's pattern an adaptation that improves output—or a distortion the nervous system is paying for in the background? That question is where predictable care begins.

JASON: WHEN THE FRAME CAN'T CARRY THE LOAD

Jason wasn't just promising; he was a phenomenon—a university hockey player whose mix of speed, aggression, and effortless torque made the jump to pro hockey look like a formality. Scouts saw what they always look for: repeatable force under fatigue, presence that doesn't fade when the game turns heavy. What matters to this book isn't his highlight reel. It's what his nervous system had to spend to produce it.

His early complaints were the kind elite athletes learn to dismiss: tightness that moved around, a leg that never felt quite "free," a stride that didn't feel as smooth as it should, recovery that took a little more effort than it seemed to take for the guys around him. Nothing that would trigger a medical alarm. Nothing that would justify a big story. In high level sport, those sensations are often treated as background noise—normal friction in a life built on load. But friction is not the same as resilience.

When I assessed him in the Vancouver Canucks training room in 1991, it was clear the issue wasn't a lack of strength or a lack of will. His body was organized around a foundation problem—not the usual sport bias you'd expect in a rotational athlete, but something more expensive: a distortion pattern that made force production possible while making force production costly. And the body always collects its fee.

Once a foundation is off, the rest of the system becomes a professional compensator. The rib cage rotates to keep the horizon level. The diaphragm starts bracing instead of moving. The upper cervical spine works overtime to keep the eyes organized under speed. Even the jaw can get recruited—not as a dental issue, but as an emergency stabilizer when the system is running out of options.

If you only look at output, that kind of athlete appears durable. If you look at cost, you see a different picture: a nervous system doing brilliant work to keep performance intact while quietly spending capacity. This is the uncomfortable clinical truth: elite performers often build their careers on the ability to compensate without looking like they're compensating. Their movement doesn't always look "bad." It can look extraordinary.

But extraordinary output can coexist with extraordinary internal load, which is why athletes so often seem to go from "fine" to "done" in a single moment. The collapse point is rarely the first time the system is challenged. It's the first time the system is challenged after capacity has already been spent—when the bucket is full and the body has no remaining tricks. That's why the same athlete can train for months and look unstoppable, then break "out of nowhere" on a routine rep, a routine sprint, a routine pivot. It was never out of nowhere. It was the first visible crack in a structure that had been held together by nervous system brilliance.

Jason wasn't fragile. He was overperforming. And in overperforming athletes, symptoms often appear late—after the body has exhausted quieter options.

WHY ATHLETES CONFUSE CLINICIANS

Athletes do two things exceptionally well that can mislead even thoughtful clinicians. First, they tolerate noise. A non-athlete experiences early warning signs as disruption. An athlete experiences the same signs as information—something to manage, ignore, or train through. Many athletes can live for years with joint irritation, altered breathing mechanics, and persistent asymmetry because they have already built an identity around functioning under stress.

Second, they create short-term stability at the expense of long-term coherence. Athletic nervous systems learn quick fixes fast: bracing, co-contraction, altered joint strategy, jaw clenching, rib rigidity, altered gait timing. These strategies are not moral failures. They are intelligent survival solutions. The problem is that survival solutions are expensive — and sport is a cash-only business.

What makes this paradox so deceptive is that the nervous system is not responding to pain. It is responding to prediction.

When the system senses that stability is uncertain—even if the athlete can still produce extraordinary output—it predicts risk and quietly increases protection. Bracing replaces fluid motion. Breathing stiffens. Muscles co-contract. The jaw tightens. The system becomes more defensive not because the athlete is weak, but because the nervous system is trying to guarantee stability under extreme load.

Elite athletes are therefore capable of performing at remarkable levels while their nervous system is already operating in a protective mode. The performance remains visible. The cost remains hidden.

Until it doesn't.

When the athlete is young, the system often has enough capacity to pay the bill. As years accumulate, that bill compounds—not because the athlete became weak, but because life and sport have been withdrawing from the same account: sleep, stress, travel, microtrauma, limited recovery windows, nutritional inconsistency, repeated sympathetic arousal, and the sheer neurological cost of performing at speed. This is why many high performers look fine on the outside while their internal organization slowly deteriorates.

It is also why "common sense" rehab advice can underperform with athletes. In a system already spending heavily, adding more demand—even demand that looks healthy on paper—can become the final straw. For clinicians, the implication is straightforward: if you evaluate the athlete the same way you evaluate the general population, you will miss the early story. You will treat overflow. You will chase symptoms. You will assume the body is failing when it is actually compensating.

The question is not, "Is the athlete strong?" The question is, "Is the athlete organized enough to keep expressing that strength without paying with breakdown?"

THE ROLE OF NON-ADVANTAGEOUS DISTORTION

A clinician must be able to distinguish two categories of asymmetry: advantageous asymmetry—rotational bias, side dominance, sport-specific patterns that improve output—and non-advantageous distortion—patterns that increase cost without improving performance.

This distinction matters for performance-minded clinicians who correctly emphasize sport-specific adaptation. The athlete does not need to be perfectly symmetrical. In some sports, symmetry would be unrealistic and performance-limiting. But no athlete benefits from distortions that degrade the system's ability to organize against gravity and transfer force cleanly: tibial torsion, genu valgum, pelvic torsion, CCJ malalignment, or a TMJ system recruited as a stabilizer. Those are not useful sport bias. They are capacity leaks.

This is where the Teeth-to-Toes model becomes less like a philosophy and more like a practical sorting tool. It helps you decide whether you are looking at a performance adaptation or an invisible tax.

ALIGNMENT IS THE EDGE

Most athletes are not limited by motivation. They are limited by mechanics and nervous system bandwidth.

Coaches tell athletes to strengthen their core, activate glutes, mobilize hips, open thoracic spine, and clean up technique. These are not wrong ideas. In the right system, at the right time, they can be excellent. But there is a catch that explains countless stubborn cases: many traditional "fixes" are attempts to add demand to a system that is already paying for non-advantageous distortion.

You cannot consistently improve output when the body is fighting its own geometry. You cannot fully restore a shoulder that is being subtly pulled off axis by a pelvis that is not transferring force cleanly. You cannot stabilize a neck that is compensating for airway compromise, rib rigidity, or pelvic distortion. You cannot create clean gait mechanics when torsion exists at the base. You cannot "relax" a jaw that has been recruited as a stabilizer. And you cannot restore recovery when the nervous system is spending its nights trying to hold the body together instead of restoring capacity.

Most people's only early exposure to the idea of connectedness in the body is the old "knee bone connected to the hip bone" song—an almost universal hint that the body behaves as a chain rather than a collection of parts. The deeper truth is more precise: the body is not merely connected. It is organized. And when one key region loses coherence, other regions do not simply "hurt." They adapt. They brace. They recruit. They protect.

This is why a Teeth-to-Toes lens matters in athletic care. It is not a rejection of local treatment. It is a refusal to treat locally in isolation when the driver is global.

KEN: A CLEAN DEMONSTRATION OF ATHLETIC LOAD

Ken's story was introduced earlier, but it belongs here because it demonstrates the athlete's paradox with almost unfair clarity.

Ken was an Olympic-level bobsleigh brakeman—explosive, powerful, and capable of producing forces most bodies will never experience. His career was built on output: force transfer, acceleration, the ability to repeatedly launch a system from stillness into violence. And yet his knees kept failing him: surgeries, rehab cycles, chronic pain, persistent limitation that never quite made sense when judged against his conditioning.

For years, the clinical narrative stayed where most narratives stay: "the knee problem." That makes sense on the surface. The knee is loud. It swells. It aches. It protests. The knee demands attention. But when Ken stood for assessment, the conclusion was difficult to ignore. His pelvis was not merely biased. It was distorted in a way that increased the cost of every stride and every training session without improving output.

This was not sport-specific asymmetry. This was a foundation that could not carry load cleanly.

Once his pelvis was corrected, the change was immediate and measurable. His gait reorganized. His knees tracked differently—more cleanly, less defensively. His breathing dropped out of the chest and back toward the diaphragm. The body stopped acting like it was constantly negotiating danger signals under the hood.

And this is the line that matters most for the skeptical clinician: Ken did not become a different athlete. He became an athlete whose system no longer needed to protect itself from its own foundation.

One sentence to keep this anchored: no amount of knee-focused rehab can fully win if the structure beneath the knee is quietly increasing load with every step.

We will return to this principle in Part II when we enter the Four Gate ways, because once you learn to see pelvic distortion as a load amplifier rather than a posture issue, many athletic mysteries stop being mysterious. Ken is not the argument that alignment is everything. Ken is the argument that alignment is one of the few variables that can change the athlete's cost of doing business immediately.

THE ATHLETE'S CLIFF

When athletes break, they often break in a way that looks sudden: the acute event, the torn tissue, the "pop," the single moment everyone remembers. But the cliff is rarely created in a single day. It is created through months or years of invisible spending.

From a Teeth-to-Toes perspective, the cliff is not the injury. The cliff is the moment the nervous system can no longer afford its strategy. That's why an athlete may keep competing with clear signs of compensation, then collapse under what appears to be a normal stress. The system was not surprised by the stress. The system was bankrupt.

If you treat only the visible injury, the athlete may return—because athletes are adaptable and determined. But if you do not address the load drivers that filled the bucket, the athlete returns to the same economics: the same spending, the same protective strategies, the same unseen cost. The body will create stability however it can, and if the foundation remains unreliable, the nervous system will continue to recruit substitutes—at the pelvis, the rib cage, the CCJ, the bite.

This is not abstract. It is testable. When you reduce load meaningfully, the system changes. When you add demand on top of unresolved distortion, the system fights.

BRIDGE TO CHAPTER SIX

Part I has been about why people get stuck: protection, load, and the predictable ways the nervous system adapts until it can no longer afford its own strategies. The athlete's paradox is simply the most dramatic version of the same story: the more capable the system, the longer it can compensate—and the harder the eventual reckoning.

Now we shift into Part II: The Four Gateways. We begin where the body begins its most consequential negotiations with gravity: the pelvis. Not because everything is pelvis-first in the universe, but because the pelvis is the mechanical hub—the place where force transfer, gait, and foundational symmetry either become efficient or become expensive.

And once you understand that distinction—efficient versus expensive —you will start seeing what you have been missing in complex cases, both athletic and non-athletic: not what hurts, but what is costing the system the most to stay upright.

That is where we go next.

PART TWO

The Four Gateways

PELVIS. CCJ. BREATH. BITE.

Systems fail at predictable junctions.

The pelvis organizes mechanical load.

The cranio-cervical junction orients the head and sensory field. The breath regulates pressure, load, and threat.

The bite influences global tension and cranial positioning.

These are not isolated regions. They are gateways. Stability at these junctions determines how well the whole system functions.

CHAPTER 6

The Pelvis

WHERE THE STORY TRULY BEGINS

Part I was about why complex cases get stuck. Not because patients are fragile, or because clinicians lack skill, but because the nervous system does what nervous systems do: it protects first, adapts second, and heals best when capacity returns.

We traced how load accumulates, how adaptation becomes compensation, how compensation can tip into overwhelm, and why high performers can carry expensive patterns longer than anyone expects.

Now, in Part II, we shift from the physics of being stuck to the anatomy of escape.

The Four Gateways are not a philosophical framework. They are the regions where chronic load most reliably concentrates—where compensation tends to organize, reinforce, and eventually defend itself. They also happen to be the places where the right intervention, at the right moment, can change the whole system fast enough that even skeptical clinicians stop debating and start measuring.

We begin with the pelvis because it is the body's primary mechanical hub: the bridge between trunk and legs, the transfer station for force, and the structure gravity interrogates with every step.

When the pelvis is centered and stable enough, the rest of the body can distribute load with far less negotiation. When it is not, everything above it becomes strategy.

And here is the inconvenient part—especially for practitioners who live "upstream" in the spine, airway, and craniofacial world:

Pelvic distortion often develops without fanfare.

Patients rarely feel it happen. They feel the workarounds: tight hip flexors, stubborn hamstrings, a low back that never quite settles, a rib cage that won't rotate cleanly, a gait that becomes subtly guarded. By the time pain announces itself, the pelvis has often been drifting for months or years, and the nervous system has been spending resources just to keep the head upright and the eyes level on top of an unstable base.

So the pelvis is not the villain.

It is usually the first witness.

This chapter is not about turning posture into a moral issue or turning anatomy into geometry trivia. It's about a clinical reality:

When the pelvis loses neutral, the system pays a tax—mechanically, neurologically, and metabolically. That tax may be affordable for a while. In some bodies, for a long while. But it is never free.

To make this concrete, we start with two stories from opposite ends of the movement spectrum—professional hockey and tai chi. Different loads. Different intentions. The same lesson.

JASON: WHEN TALENT ISN'T ENOUGH

Jason belonged to a rare category of athlete: the kind everyone expects to reshape the sport. A record-setting university defenseman and a first-round NHL draft pick, his size, skill, and intelligence positioned him for dominance.

You met him in the last chapter, but he reappears here because he is one of the cleanest examples I've ever seen of a pelvis acting as the Primary Driver—quietly shaping everything until the cost becomes undeniable.

He was an elite athlete, but he could not escape one truth: He was skating on a crooked foundation.

His symptoms were subtle at first—tightness, fatigue, a sense that his stride wasn't as efficient as it should be. Nothing dramatic. Nothing unusual for a young player entering the NHL. The problem was that the compensations were accumulating, and with each passing month the inefficiency became more expensive.

At that level, "a little bit off" is not a small thing.

It's a multiplier.

When I assessed him, the answer was written clearly in his structure. His pelvis wasn't merely rotated; it was locked into a torsion pattern no amount of strength, grit, or conditioning could compensate for indefinitely. One ilium pitched forward while the other drew backward.

His lumbar spine had to negotiate the imbalance. His rib cage counterrotated to keep head position coherent. Even his stride mechanics—something coaches and players often treat as "skill"—were being steered by a distortion he never felt developing.

Jason didn't fail his body. His body did what bodies do: it protected the outcome at the cost of the system.

And to be clear, this is not an argument against sport-specific asymmetry. Many elite performances are built on side dominance and rotational bias. The concern is non-advantageous distortion—patterns that raise the cost of doing business without improving output.

No athlete benefits from tibial torsion, genu valgum, pelvic torsion, CCJ malalignment, or a TMJ system recruited as a stabilizer. Those are not performance adaptations. They are load.

This is also where pelvic distortion becomes confusing for patients: the same crooked foundation can express itself as wildly different "diagnoses," depending on where the system finally runs out of options.

Chronic back pain (as you'll see in a moment with Bill). Debilitating hip pain (like Rachel).

Knee dysfunction (like Ken).

And, in Jason's world, a sports hernia—an end-stage bill for a long-running compensation strategy that finally became too expensive to maintain.

Straightening a pelvis like Jason's doesn't merely change "posture." It changes force transfer, timing, and the neuromuscular conversation between the feet and the brain.

Jason's story is not primarily about injury.

It is about the cost of an unseen foundation—paid over thousands of reps, until the bill arrives.

BILL: THE TAI CHI INSTRUCTOR

Bill was the opposite of Jason. Not explosive. Not fast. A tai chi instructor whose discipline revolves around grace, symmetry, flow, and control.

His problem wasn't impact. It wasn't heavy load. It wasn't trauma. It was instruction.

For years, he had been taught—incorrectly—to maintain a posterior pelvic tilt as a default posture: a tucked pelvis, a "protected" spine, a shape that can feel stable in the short term.

But what feels stable is not always what is sustainable.

Over time that chronic posterior tilt became a long-term distortion. His lumbar spine flattened. The hip complex lost mechanical advantage. His glutes behaved like overworked stabilizers rather than responsive engines. The diaphragm lost freedom because the rib cage could no longer move well over the pelvis. Breath migrated upward. And the nervous system, trying to maintain balance inside a borrowed shape, began to fatigue.

The result was predictable: chronic low back pain, hip stiffness, and neck tension.

When Bill's pelvis was restored closer to neutral, the change was immediate—not because tai chi failed him, and not because movement betrayed him. He had simply trained himself into misalignment and then performed every movement inside distorted geometry.

Elegant movement performed inside a poor reference system does not become corrective.

It becomes well-practiced compensation.

Bill teaches a different lesson than Jason, but one equally important: You do not need massive force to distort the pelvis.

You only need repetition inside the wrong shape.

WHY THE PELVIS IS OFTEN THE FIRST DOMINO

Jason and Bill could not be more different. An NHL defenseman and a tai chi instructor live at opposite ends of the movement spectrum. Yet the mechanism beneath their symptoms was identical: a pelvis that drifted off neutral, and a nervous system that reorganized everything else to keep life moving forward.

This is where the old children's song—"the knee bone connected to the hip bone"—is both right and misleading. It's right in the most basic sense: the bones are connected. But it's misleading because it suggests simple linkage, like a chain.

The body is not a chain.

It is a negotiation with gravity—managed moment to moment by a nervous system that prioritizes orientation and safety over symmetry and efficiency.

When the pelvis drifts, the spine doesn't "compensate" like a passive structure. It adapts actively. The rib cage rotates to preserve head position. The diaphragm adjusts to the rib cage and pelvis it is anchored to. Tone rises where clarity is lost.

Over time, the body can begin spending more energy bracing than moving—often without the patient (or clinician) realizing that this shift has been underway for years.

That is the hidden architecture of chronic pain.

And this is why the pelvis matters so much in a Teeth-to-Toes framework. The pelvis is not just a load-bearing structure. It is an orientation signal.

When it drifts, the whole body reorganizes around it. People rarely notice the drift. They notice the downstream consequences once the cost becomes too high: the hip that seizes, the knee that becomes chronically irritated, the headaches that refuse to leave, the jaw that clenches without permission, or the neck that feels older than the rest of the body.

The pelvis is not the villain.

It is the first witness.

And if you learn to listen to it, the map of dysfunction becomes legible.

THE INVISIBLE PRESSURE

Once you recognize the pelvis as an orientation signal—not merely a set of bones—you begin to see why pelvic distortion is so costly.

The body does not simply "tilt" and carry on. It reorganizes.

A rotated or torsioned pelvis changes how the femurs load. That changes how the knees track. That changes how the feet contact the ground. The rib cage then counter-rotates to keep the eyes level and the vestibular system calm. The diaphragm adapts to the rib cage. Breath mechanics change. Tone rises. The spine becomes a mediator between competing demands instead of a conduit for efficient movement.

And because compensation is often effective, the patient usually presents late—when the nervous system is no longer paying the tax quietly.

This is also why pelvic correction, when it is real and stabilized, can be dramatic. It doesn't simply "improve posture." It reduces global negotiation. It gives the system a cleaner reference point. It lowers the baseline demand required just to stand, walk, sit, and breathe.

But a thoughtful clinician should pause here and avoid a new oversimplification.

The body is not built like a stack of blocks. It behaves more like a tensegrity structure—a system where stability comes from balanced tension, not rigid pieces sitting neatly on top of one another. Change tension in one region and the whole shape reorganizes.

That's why a pelvis that drifts doesn't simply create a "pelvic problem." It changes the tension map everywhere: the rib cage stiffens to substitute for stability, the diaphragm braces to control motion it can't trust, the upper neck works overtime to keep the horizon level, and even the jaw can be recruited as a last-resort stabilizer.

In a tensegrity system, the question is rarely "Where does it hurt?"

The better question is: Where did the structure lose balance—and what did the nervous system have to tighten to keep you upright?

The pelvis is the mechanical gateway, and in many cases it is the first domino. Yet the body does not serve the pelvis as its highest priority.

The body serves the head.

The nervous system will sacrifice symmetry, efficiency, and comfort to keep the head oriented in space. It will torque the rib cage, brace the diaphragm, and—when necessary—recruit the jaw as a stabilizer if that is what it takes to keep the eyes level and the world tolerable.

We'll return to this principle later, because it explains a pattern every experienced clinician has seen: a correction that looks clean in isolation but won't hold in the real world until another gateway is addressed.

Which brings us to the next chapter.

BRIDGE TO CHAPTER SEVEN

If the pelvis is the mechanical hub, the cranio-cervical junction is the neurological one—where head orientation, vestibular input, visual calibration, protective reflexes, and proprioceptive clarity converge.

When the CCJ is off enough to create confusion—or when the nervous system no longer trusts the head's position in space—compensation propagates everywhere, including back down into the rib cage and pelvis.

In the chapter ahead, we'll look at the CCJ not as a niche specialty topic, but as a foundational gateway in complex chronic pain: a region whose influence is often underestimated until you see what happens when it's stabilized properly.

That is where we go next.

CHAPTER 7

The CCJ

THE CONTROL TOWER

In the previous chapter we established the pelvis as the mechanical hub: the structure that transfers load between trunk and legs, and the place where many long-term compensation patterns quietly begin.

But there is an equally important truth—one that explains why some pelvic corrections don't hold, why some patients remain globally guarded despite doing "all the right things," and why a few millimetres at the top of the spine can change the entire tone of the system.

If the pelvis is the foundation, the cranio-cervical junction is the compass.

At the top of the spine—between the base of the skull and the first two vertebrae—lives one of the most powerful and misunderstood regions in human biomechanics: the cranio-cervical junction, or CCJ. This is not simply a joint that "holds up the head." Functionally, it behaves more like a high-density sensorimotor integration zone—an interface where mechanical reality becomes neurological governance, where the body decides how vigilant it needs to be just to exist inside gravity.

When the pelvis drifts, the body can often negotiate the distortion for a long time. When the CCJ loses clarity, the nervous system often changes its entire posture of engagement.

That's why the CCJ earns the metaphor: the control tower.

ORIENTATION IS A SURVIVAL PROBLEM, NOT A POSTURE PROBLEM

Long before the jaw begins to strain, long before the bite fractures sensory clarity, and long before breath rises into the upper ribs and refuses to descend, something quieter can begin to shift: the orientation system.

The nervous system is relentlessly concerned with a few non-negotiables: Where is "up"? Where is the horizon? Where is my head in space? Is my airway secure? Is balance stable enough to move without threat?

The CCJ is where these questions become actionable. It's where the body's insistence on orientation becomes physical strategy—tone, bracing, rib stiffness, jaw recruitment, pelvic rotation—anything, anywhere, as long as the head stays coherent enough for the world to feel tolerable.

This is why the CCJ is rarely the only issue, yet so often becomes the loudest one. When the foundation is off, the system can sometimes compensate. When the control tower is off, the system tends to become vigilant.

And vigilance is expensive.

WHY THIS TINY JOINT HAS OUTSIZED INFLUENCE

One reason the CCJ can change the whole system is that it isn't built like the rest of the spine. The atlas (C1) has no disc. The axis (C2) houses the dens—a precision peg the nervous system treats like sacred architecture. Major arteries pass through this region. The lower brainstem lives here. Key regulatory nerves emerge here. The ligaments are designed for accuracy, not brute force.

In plain language: the CCJ is engineered for stability with micro-movement, not big sloppy motion. That's why small deviations can produce large consequences. At this level, millimetres matter. Angles matter. Symmetry matters.

There's a moment Dr. Jeff Scholten describes that captures biological hierarchy without turning it into a turf war. Years ago, the night before a dental conference, he found himself in a lively debate with a group of dentists arguing—passionately and intelligently—that the TMJ might be the most important joint in the body.

When they finished, Jeff smiled and asked a simple, brutal question:

"If you take a bullet to the TMJ or the CCJ... which one is worse?"

Silence.

The point wasn't to "win." It was to reveal the hierarchy the body already lives by. The TMJ matters—sometimes enormously—because the bite is a powerful neurological input and a stabilizer for the head–neck system. But the CCJ sits closer to the non-negotiable the nervous system will protect at any cost: the brainstem and the machinery that keeps you alive.

Orientation is a survival problem. So is circulation. So is airway control. And the CCJ lives at the crossroads of all three.

That's why the body will distort everything downstream to protect it. It will recruit jaw tension, elevate global tone, rotate the rib cage, twist the pelvis, and sacrifice comfort anywhere it has to—because if stability fails at the control tower, the priority isn't "good posture."

It's survival.

WHERE SENSATION BECOMES POSITION

The CCJ contains one of the densest concentrations of proprioceptors anywhere in the spine. In plain language, it's loaded with sensors whose job is to feed the brainstem and cerebellum continuous information about orientation, balance, eye position, airway strategy, and postural tone.

This is one of the most useful reframes in the Teeth-to-Toes model: the CCJ is less a mechanical hinge and more a neurological reference system.

When reference systems are clean, the nervous system spends less energy protecting. When reference systems become noisy—whether from a distorted pelvis, an unstable atlas, airway compromise, or a mismatched bite—the body reorganizes around uncertainty. Tone rises. Breath changes. Movement stiffens. Compensation becomes reflexive.

Symptoms can show up in forms that frustrate conventional thinking: headaches, dizziness, jaw fatigue, balance disturbance, unexplained fatigue, altered breathing patterns, persistent asymmetry, and a neck that never feels truly settled.

Imaging may be unrevealing—not because nothing is happening, but because the primary issue is often not damage.

It's distorted information and the protective strategies that follow.

That distinction matters, because it changes what we aim to restore. We're not chasing looseness. We're chasing clarity.

TENSEGRITY REMINDER: WHEN THE TENT GETS LOUD

In Chapter Six we talked about tensegrity—how the body behaves less like a stack of blocks and more like a tent: stability comes from balanced tension, not rigid pieces.

The CCJ is one of the places where that tent "talks" the loudest.

When the CCJ is neutral, muscular effort often drops, tension distributes more evenly, and movement can feel lighter—as though the body has stopped arguing with itself about where it is in space.

When the CCJ is off, reflexive tension increases, breathing often becomes shallower, the spine twists to keep the eyes level, and the pelvis adapts.

The system gets louder—not because you're weak, but because the body is solving an orientation problem it does not feel safe ignoring.

THE THREE TYPES OF TIGHTNESS — ONLY ONE REALLY MATTERS

There's a distinction Dr. Scholten teaches that rewires how you interpret "tight muscles."

First is active tightness: you worked hard, you lifted something heavy, you spent the weekend hunched over a project you'll pretend was fun. The muscle is sore and tight because it was used. That's normal.

Second is habitual tightness: the posture you live in becomes the posture you own. Long hours sitting, repetitive tasks, a favored stance at the kitchen counter—patterns that become default settings.

But the third type is the one that derails complex cases: reflexive tightness. This is not a muscle problem. It's a protection problem.

When the head is subtly off-centre, when the CCJ loses clarity, the nervous system reads uncertainty where it most hates uncertainty—at the control tower. And when orientation feels threatened, the body doesn't negotiate.

It braces.

Tone rises. The neck, jaw, rib cage, and even the hips can behave like they're in a low-grade emergency, because the system is trying to keep the eyes level and the world tolerable.

Here's the part that matters clinically and personally: you can't stretch your way out of reflexive tightness. You can't massage your way out of it. You can't strengthen your way out of it.

Those inputs may feel good temporarily, but they often don't hold—because the driver is still online.

Restore CCJ clarity, and something almost unfair can happen: the tension that looked stubborn suddenly behaves like it was never the real problem.

That distinction changes outcomes not because it adds a new technique, but because it prevents clinicians from treating a symptom as though it were a cause.

Upper cervical care stops sounding like "neck work" and starts making sense as what it often is at its best: a precision attempt to restore orientation so the whole system can finally stop defending.

A QUIET PIECE OF THE PUZZLE: RECOVERY AND CLEARANCE

Here is a newer piece of the conversation that deserves a patient-facing translation, because it reinforces something experienced clinicians have sensed for a long time: long-term brain health depends, in part, on whether the brain can clear its own metabolic waste efficiently—especially during deeper, restorative sleep. Researchers often call this the glymphatic system.

You don't need the vocabulary. You need the idea: recovery isn't only about rest. It's also about clearance.

I'm not bringing this up to make claims we can't prove at the individual level. I'm bringing it up because it widens the frame. The CCJ may matter not only because it influences pain, posture, and balance—but because it can influence the conditions under which the brain recovers.

Even if you ignore every technical term, the clinical point still holds: when orientation is noisy and vigilance stays high, sleep quality tends to drop, breathing stays guarded, tone stays elevated, and the system's ability to reset gets weaker.

A control tower that can't find the horizon doesn't just affect movement. It can affect recovery.

WHY THE CCJ BECOMES OVERLOADED WHEN THE PELVIS TWISTS

When the pelvis rotates, tilts, or spirals, it forces the spine into compensatory geometry. The CCJ becomes the final hinge the body uses to keep the head upright and the visual horizon level.

A crooked pelvis doesn't merely change low back mechanics. It often increases the workload on the CCJ—more rotational demand, more bracing, more protective tone, more vigilance.

This is why so many patients with pelvic torsion present with a familiar cluster: chronic neck stiffness, headaches, jaw fatigue, restricted head rotation, the sense that the neck is always working, or subtle instability high in the spine.

The CCJ is not failing.

It is doing its job—compensating for a foundation that can't fully support it.

At the same time, a complete model has to allow for the inverse. Sometimes the pelvis is reacting to the CCJ.

WHEN THE CCJ IS THE PRIMARY DRIVER

In many complex chronic pain cases, pelvic asymmetry is the first driver you can see. But not always. Occasionally the CCJ is the first domino—the region that destabilizes orientation so profoundly that the rest of the body, including the pelvis, organizes around it.

Here is a simple example from a Teeth-to-Toes training session.

Standing, a dentist we assessed displayed clear pelvic asymmetry: the left side sat higher than the right, though her pelvic tilt looked symmetrical and comfortably within a healthy range. I expected to find the most common pattern beneath weightbearing pelvic asymmetry—a functionally short leg, the right leg in this case. However, when she lay down her lower body became remarkably symmetrical. No functional leg-length difference.

That shift was too clean to ignore.

So we performed the Cervical Syndrome Test. Turning her head to the left made her left leg shorten instantly. Turning her head to the right equalized her leg lengths again.

In under two minutes, the hierarchy revealed itself. Her pelvis wasn't leading the pattern.

Her neck was.

This doesn't mean the bite is irrelevant. It doesn't mean the pelvis will never need attention. It means something much more practical: if you want her results to hold, the CCJ must be addressed early enough in her sequence that the nervous system stops fighting for orientation.

We'll return to this idea later, because it is one of the most reliable reasons "good work" fails to persist: the correct intervention, delivered to the wrong driver, at the wrong moment.

THE HIDDEN MULTIPLIER: FORWARD HEAD LOAD AND THE THREAT BUCKET

The Threat Bucket chapter gave you a framework that becomes concrete at the CCJ. Head position is not merely a cosmetic posture issue. When the head drifts forward of the body's midline, the mechanical demand on the neck rises sharply—and the neurological demand rises with it.

The body has no choice but to respond. The Righting Reflex fires. The CCJ tightens its grip on orientation. Muscles brace. Tone rises.

This is why small changes at the CCJ can have outsized effects: a few millimetres of drift can raise global tone; a few millimetres of restored orientation can reduce the system's need to protect—not because we "fixed the neck," but because we reduced confusion.

ARCHITECTURE VERSUS ADAPTATION

Every so often the body reminds us that alignment is not solely a matter of habit. There are quiet anatomical variations—differences in the shape of the atlas, the occiput, joint surfaces, or connective tissue behavior—that may never matter in typical life, but can become consequential under collision, cumulative load, or sustained compensatory demand.

These variations don't make a person fragile. They make them individual.

Here is the clinically useful distinction: structural asymmetry sets the baseline; functional asymmetry determines the trajectory. One is the blueprint you inherit. The other is the story your nervous system writes in response to the world.

The CCJ sits at the crossroads of both, which is why it can be subtle on imaging and profound in lived physiology.

THE "YES-LOOP": WHEN THE BODY REINFORCES ITS OWN PATTERN

Dr. Scholten describes a loop we see constantly: a small imbalance up top recruits compensation below, and the compensation below feeds right back into the imbalance up top.

Patients often describe it perfectly without knowing the mechanics: "I get temporary relief, but it never holds," or "Everything feels connected, but I can't explain how."

Of course it feels that way. The loop is still running.

The clinical goal is not to chase every symptom. It's to find the driver that keeps the loop active and reduce it enough that the system can stop pulling itself back into the same groove.

When that happens, people tend to describe it the same way: "My body stopped fighting itself." "My breathing opened." "Standing feels easier."

Not magic. Just a system finally getting a cleaner answer.

SEAN: WHEN THE CONTROL TOWER LOSES ITS BEARINGS

Sean's case, introduced earlier, is a clean example of what happens when the control tower itself becomes unstable. His nervous system could no longer maintain reliable orientation. Symptoms multiplied. Reactivity escalated. Downstream interventions could help briefly, but nothing could hold because the system lacked a stable reference point to organize around.

His recovery was not a dramatic fix. It was the slow, precise return of tolerable orientation: upper cervical correction and monitoring, careful reassessment, appropriately dosed manual work and corrective exercise, and a pace his nervous system could deal with.

We'll return to Sean later as well, because cases like his teach restraint—one of the most underrated clinical skills in chronic pain work. When the control tower is unstable, the goal is not to add more inputs. It's to reduce threat, restore clarity, and let the system accept change without flaring into defense.

WHAT UPPER CERVICAL CARE IS—AND WHAT IT IS NOT

It's worth being explicit here, because the CCJ attracts both skepticism and overenthusiasm.

Precision-based upper cervical work—NUCCA care is one example—is not a mobility program and not a forceful attempt to free up the neck. At its best, it is a neurological recalibration aimed at restoring orientation rather than chasing range of motion.

The intent is not to make the neck looser, but to make the nervous system quieter so the body can reestablish midline, balance, and reflexive stability on its own.

When addressed at the right moment in a case, this can reduce neurological load dramatically. When addressed too early—while destabilizing forces below remain unchanged—it may not hold. When addressed too late, the system may remain trapped in vigilance.

Correct it at the right moment, and the nervous system often reorganizes with a precision that feels almost unfair to anyone still arguing that mechanics don't matter.

Patients rarely describe this as "my pain went away first." They describe something more diagnostic: relief, calm, orientation—a sense that the body has remembered where "up" is again.

WHY THIS CHAPTER POINTS TOWARD DENTISTRY WITHOUT TRYING TO BE DENTISTRY

This is also where Dr. Curtis Westersund enters the conversation. Even excellent CCJ work can struggle to hold if the bite is feeding distortion back into the head–neck system. A high crown, an uneven restoration, or a subtle shift in how the jaw finds home can change cranial strain patterns and make the CCJ work harder than it should.

That doesn't mean dentistry is always first or always last. It means the jaw and the CCJ often behave like partners.

Upper cervical work helps stabilize the head–neck axis. Functional dentistry helps stabilize the mandible–cranium relationship. Together, they give the nervous system its best chance to stay organized.

We'll return to that partnership later, because it helps explain something patients and clinicians both find maddening: why a correction can look perfect in isolation—and still fail to hold if another gateway is quietly distorting the signal.

BRIDGE TO THE NEXT GATEWAY: THE BREATH

If the pelvis is the mechanical hub and the CCJ is the orientation hub, the breath is the regulatory hub—the interface between structure and autonomic state.

The diaphragm doesn't simply move air. It coordinates rib mechanics, spinal stabilization, pressure management, and nervous system tone. When orientation is threatened, breath becomes defensive. When breath stays defensive, it becomes a chronic load generator.

In the next chapter we'll look at breathing not as a wellness trend, but as a clinical gateway: how rib cage mechanics, diaphragm behavior, airway strategy, and nervous system state either drain the bucket—or keep filling it.

That is where we go next.

CHAPTER 8

The Breath

REGULATING PRESSURE, LOAD, AND THREAT

If the previous chapter showed how the cranio-cervical junction tells the body where "up" is, this chapter shows something just as useful: how the body signals whether it believes that orientation is safe.

Breath is the nervous system's most honest dashboard light.

Most clinicians were trained to treat breathing as background—important, of course, but rarely central unless we're talking about lungs, asthma, or conditioning. Complex chronic pain teaches a different lesson. Watch enough of these cases unfold and breath stops looking like a passive reflex and starts looking like an organizing strategy: one of the ways the system manages load, threat, and stability when it can't do so quietly anymore.

In complex patients, you can debate almost anything—until you can't. Eventually the case forces you to confront the same two amplifiers again and again: the jaw and the breath.

Kelly Starrett summed this up: "Everyone that knows gets to the jaw and breathing eventually." He wasn't being poetic. He was describing what you see when you stop treating symptoms as isolated events and start treating them as outputs of a whole system under load.

BREATH IS NOT BACKGROUND

Breath is not neutral. Breath is not random. Breath reflects state.

A patient can walk into a clinic with a calm voice and a tidy history and still be breathing as if they're about to be tackled. And a patient can arrive with a long list of symptoms and—when they finally exhale fully—you can often see the nervous system loosen its grip on the day, as though the body had been holding its breath against life and has suddenly found permission to set it down.

This is why breath matters so much in a Teeth-to-Toes model. It's the one movement your nervous system never stops negotiating. It happens when you're conscious and when you're not. It happens in pain and in peace. It happens under load, in fear, in sleep debt, and in the micro-moments where the system decides whether to brace or soften.

Because it's continuous, it's revealing.

Breath often tells the truth before the patient has words for it. And it often changes before the patient reports that anything has changed.

THE "DEM BONES" PROBLEM

Most intelligent people have almost no formal exposure to whole-body interdependence. Their universal entry point is childhood logic: the knee bone linked to the thigh bone, the thigh bone linked to the hip bone—and a catchy song that implies the body is a neat chain of parts.

Clinical reality is messier and more interesting. The body isn't merely connected; it's coordinated. It's a living system whose job is to negotiate gravity, keep the head oriented, protect the airway, and distribute load without triggering threat.

When coordination is efficient, breath is quiet and deep.

When coordination is strained, breath becomes compensation—sometimes the compensation.

THE AIRWAY'S LONG SHADOW

Breath can't be understood without respecting airway development.

Some people begin life with an airway operating near the edge of its capacity. Genetics can set the stage—narrow palates, retruded jaws, crowded teeth—but development often determines whether that stage becomes a long-term performance problem for the nervous system.

When nasal breathing is compromised early, mouth breathing becomes the workaround. Mouth breathing changes tongue posture. Tongue posture influences palate shape. Palate shape influences the bite. The bite influences cranial strain. Cranial strain influences upper cervical orientation. Upper cervical orientation influences rib mechanics. Rib mechanics determine whether the diaphragm moves freely—or braces like armor.

By adulthood, the person rarely identifies any of this as "an airway story." They simply report patterns clinicians recognize immediately once they know to look: shoulders living too close to ears, a neck that never feels off-duty, a jaw that behaves like a clamp, a rib cage that doesn't expand well posteriorly, and a breath that never seems to drop.

Breath told the truth years before pain was given the microphone.

We'll return to the bite soon, because it isn't merely "teeth meeting teeth." It's a sensory-organizing system that can either clarify the skull and neck—or destabilize them.

WHY SHALLOW BREATHING KEEPS THE THREAT SYSTEM ONLINE

When the system is overloaded, breathing strategy often changes. It becomes faster, shallower, and more upper-chest dominant. Clinically, this is often labeled "anxiety breathing," but that language can mislead, because it implies the cause is psychological.

In many patients, it's mechanical and neurophysiologic before it's emotional: restricted ribs, a guarded diaphragm, a forward head pattern, a CCJ under demand, a jaw recruited as a stabilizer, and a nervous system that has learned to live in readiness.

Over time, a shallow, defensive breathing pattern keeps the stress-response machinery easier to trigger and harder to shut off. The system receives fewer internal "green lights" of safety—full exhalation, comfortable rib motion, diaphragmatic excursion, and the downshifting that tends to follow them.

Sleep fragments. Recovery slows. Reactivity rises. What clinicians call sensitization is experienced by the patient as a whole-body state—loud, tiring, and hard to escape.

This matters because chronic pain is rarely a single tissue problem. It's often a state problem.

And breath is one of the most sensitive readouts of that state.

BREATH AS A CLINICAL METRIC

Patients often ask, "How do I know I'm getting better?"

Breath often answers earlier than symptoms do.

When the ribs soften, when the exhale lengthens without coaching, when the shoulders drop, when the jaw stops bracing between words, when the diaphragm moves without guarding, when the patient stops needing to "remember" to breathe—those aren't vague wellness markers. They're evidence that the nervous system is spending less of its budget on vigilance.

This is why breath is such a useful retest variable in complex cases. It changes with load. It changes with orientation. It changes with threat. It changes with sequence. And it often relapses early when the system is pushed too hard, too fast, or in the wrong order.

Breath doesn't lie.

And, to borrow a line I've heard Javier Vasquez use in a way every experienced clinician understands: you know something real is shifting "when the patient starts breathing like a horse"—grounded, unmistakably diaphragmatic, and impossible to fake. Not elegant. Not polite. Honest.

There's another reason breath matters that most people never hear in a rehab setting: your brain has a nightly clean-up job. While you sleep—especially when sleep is deep—the body does housekeeping. It clears metabolic clutter, resets sensitivity, and restores the bandwidth you burn through all day just being a human under gravity.

That clean-up shift doesn't run well when the nervous system is stuck in fight-or-flight. If you're braced, clenching, shallow-breathing, and scanning for danger, sleep gets lighter. You wake up tired. And the next day the system is easier to trigger—not because you're broken, but because you didn't get the recovery you were supposed to get.

This is why breath is such a reliable marker. When breath drops lower, when the exhale lengthens, when you feel that unforced "ahhh" happen on its own, the system is doing something deeper than relaxing.

It is shifting into a state where repair is finally allowed.

BREATH AS A TOOL

Breath isn't only a diagnostic mirror. It can also be used as a gentle lever—if we respect state.

The mistake clinicians sometimes make is asking for "good breathing" too early, as if a patient with a guarded diaphragm and rigid ribs can simply will their way into parasympathetic tone.

When the system is overloaded, demanding breathwork can backfire. It can provoke light-headedness, anxiety, chest tightness, or a sense of internal alarm—not because breathing is harmful, but because the nervous system interprets the demand as threat.

So we start simple. We choose patterns that are rhythmic, tolerable, and forgiving—patterns that invite downshifting without forcing performance. In many patients, a steady cadence with a gentle pause is enough to begin changing tone. The goal isn't mastery.

The goal is capacity: enough stability that the system can tolerate deeper structural work and more specific retraining.

Later—when the ribs move better, when the diaphragm is less defensive, when orientation is clearer—we can use more potent patterns strategically. Longer exhales, longer pauses, and more deliberate nasal breathing can become powerful tools, not because they're magic, but because the nervous system is finally able to interpret them as safe.

This is where the Teeth-to-Toes principle shows up again: breathwork is dosage and timing. The same tool can organize in one state and destabilize in another.

HOW THE GATEWAYS TALK TO EACH OTHER

Breath depends on structure. Structure depends on orientation. Orientation depends on load. Load is managed by the nervous system.

Straighten the pelvis and breath often changes immediately. Stabilize the CCJ and breathing strategy frequently settles. Restore rib motion and the diaphragm becomes less defensive. Improve airway function and breath drops without being coached. Clarify the bite and upstream tone patterns can soften.

Breath is rarely the root cause. Breath is often the reflection.

And it's often the first reflection to normalize when you're finally working in the right order.

BRIDGE TO THE BITE

This chapter isn't about perfect breathing. It's about reclaiming breath as a clinical signal—and a patient-accessible metric you can monitor in real time, in any room, on any day.

But there is a structure that can disrupt breathing strategy without changing a single rib angle, and can amplify CCJ demand without a dramatic "neck injury." It can alter cranial strain patterns in microns, not degrees, and recruit the jaw into the postural system so quietly that neither patient nor clinician recognizes it at first.

That structure is the bite.

That is where we go next.

CHAPTER 9

The Bite

WHEN MILLIMETRES BECOME BIOLOGY

By the time most people reach the bite, they've already lived through every other kind of explanation. They've been told it's their core, their discs, their stress, their age, their posture, their mindset, their "weak glutes," or their "tight hip flexors." They've tried treatment that helped briefly, and they've tried treatment that did nothing at all.

What they rarely hear—early enough—is that one of the smallest mechanical regions in the body can influence one of the largest governing systems: the cranial, cervical, respiratory, and postural network that decides how safe it is to exist inside gravity.

So let's define terms, because "bite" gets misunderstood even inside dentistry.

The bite includes how your teeth meet, but it isn't merely the pattern of tooth contact on a piece of paper. It is also the neurological information your brain receives from that contact—through exquisitely sensitive receptors in the teeth, periodontal ligaments, jaw muscles, and the joints themselves.

In other words, the bite is a reference system. It helps the nervous system answer questions it cares about far more than aesthetics: Where is my mandible? How stable is my head? Is my airway safe? Is clenching required to feel organized? Can I downshift?

That's why bite isn't "just dentistry," and why this chapter matters even if you've never had braces, never worn a night guard, and have never once complained about your teeth.

A few millimetres of vertical height. A slight shift in mandibular position. A barely perceptible torque in the jaw.

Those aren't cosmetic details. They are sensory events—signals the nervous system may interpret as orientation cues, airway cues, threat cues, or relief cues. And because the bite sits at the crossroads of airway strategy, cranial strain patterns, jaw mechanics, and upper-cervical stability, even tiny distortions can echo through the entire body.

Here is the quiet truth most people don't hear until they've paid for it:

The bite is rarely the beginning of the story, yet it is often the structure that decides how the story ends.

Three patients show the spectrum of what the bite can do to a body—when it destabilizes, when it is mistimed, and when it finally integrates: Raji, Julie, and Kim.

RAJI: WHEN DENTISTRY WAS THE FIRST DOMINO

If you want a clean demonstration of how powerful the bite can be, start with the case where it clearly led the pattern.

Raji's story began with a cosmetic makeover—elective, routine, well-intentioned. What followed was not routine. The work left her with a profoundly dysfunctional bite, and while we don't need to speculate about which single detail caused which symptom, we do know this: her system changed after the procedure. Not all at once, and not always dramatically, but relentlessly—like a weather front that never quite moves on.

Her new bite triggered a cascade that looked "unrelated" on paper, yet was brutally consistent in real life: cranial strain, cervical tension, ribcage rotation, altered breathing strategy, pelvic torsion, groin pain, hip instability, gait distortion, chronic neurological overload, and a threat bucket that never seemed to empty.

The body didn't merely develop symptoms. It adopted a new operating strategy—one built around stabilizing uncertainty.

One underappreciated part of that cascade was hypervigilance—not as psychology, but as physiology. In some bodies, especially hypermobile ones, the jaw and upper neck become high-stakes reference points. When passive stability is low and sensory clarity is unreliable, the nervous system compensates by monitoring more. It doesn't relax into autopilot. It runs on scanning.

In Raji's case, hypervigilance wasn't "worry." It was survival logic. When the nervous system can't find a reliable reference point, it stops trusting the background and starts policing the foreground. Tooth contact becomes a coordinate system. Jaw position becomes a threat assessment. Sleep gets lighter. Small changes feel bigger than they should. Clenching becomes less a habit than a stabilizing strategy—an unconscious attempt to manufacture certainty in a system that no longer trusts its own input.

If you remember the Threat Bucket, this is what it looks like when the system can't find "stable."

By the time she sought help, she was years into the pattern—battling symptoms no one connected back to the dental work that started it all. Her recovery has been long, complex, and still unfolding. There was no single correction that lifted her out. She has required upper cervical care, dental stabilization, corrective exercise, breathwork, persistence, and more time than she ever expected.

And here is the uncomfortable truth Raji forces us to face: not every case ends in perfect silence. In long-standing, load-sensitive systems, the goal is sometimes not a cinematic resolution, but a quieter baseline, fewer storms, shorter storms, and a body that becomes more predictable again.

That is not a consolation prize. That is the nervous system regaining capacity—slowly, and sometimes reluctantly—after years of running in protection.

Raji teaches the first lesson of this chapter:

When the bite destabilizes the system early, everything downstream pays.

JULIE: WHEN "EARLY" MADE IT WORSE

Julie's story teaches the next lesson: even when dentistry is relevant, timing can turn a good idea into a destabilizing one.

When her dentist attempted to adjust her bite early in her journey, her jaw locked—sometimes for ten hours at a time. That isn't "a failure of dentistry." That is a nervous system rejecting an input it cannot safely integrate.

The jaw wasn't being dramatic. It was being loyal. It was doing what the body does when the ground beneath it feels unstable: it grabs.

In a load-sensitive system, a bite change can behave like an earthquake. If the base is unstable, if the CCJ is already compensating, if breath is defensive, if the threat bucket is full, even a small occlusal change can provoke a protective storm.

In hindsight, it wasn't just her jaw reacting. It was her whole system rejecting uncertainty and escalating into protection.

This is where good intent becomes insufficient. In complex cases, the question isn't merely what you do. It's when you do it.

Julie's case also carries an important warning: when a system is overloaded, it can mislead the clinician. Early dental work may appear to "fail" because the bite doesn't matter. But sometimes it fails because the bite matters too much—because the nervous system is already using it as a stabilizer while everything beneath it is still moving.

Julie teaches the second lesson:

A bite intervention delivered too early can increase threat—because the system cannot stabilize around a moving platform.

KIM: WHEN THE BITE WAS THE FINAL PIECE

Kim's story is the counterweight. It shows what can happen when the sequence is respected—when the system becomes coherent enough to tell the truth, and stable enough to accept the final input.

Her trouble didn't begin with dentistry. It began with trauma: a motor-vehicle accident, immediate neck strain, jaw rigidity, dizziness, headaches, cognitive fog—the unmistakable signature of a nervous system pushed beyond its capacity.

She found meaningful help early through excellent upper cervical care. Not perfectly and not completely, but enough to keep her afloat.

When she arrived at our clinic, we assessed her from the ground up. Her pelvis needed correction. Her posture needed to become more organized. Her system needed a cleaner mechanical reference point so her nervous system could stop spending so much bandwidth simply staying upright.

Those changes helped—substantially. Her protective bracing eased. Her baseline improved.

But she didn't cross the finish line.

That moment teaches one of the deepest lessons in complex cases: improvement isn't the same as resolution, and "better" isn't proof you've found the true limiting factor.

In Kim's case, it took time—and teamwork—to realize that even as the base became more stable, something upstream remained incompatible with the body she was becoming.

It wasn't her back. It wasn't her pelvis. It wasn't even primarily her neck.

It was her bite.

Here is what often happens in long-standing compensation: the bite adapts to the best available version of the body. If that body has been twisted, guarded, and neurologically defensive for years, the bite may settle into a position that works for survival inside that distortion.

When you begin restoring the system beneath it—when the pelvis straightens and the upper cervical region quiets—the bite may no longer match the new organization.

The old bite wasn't "wrong" in a moral or cosmetic sense. It was simply the best the nervous system could do under the circumstances.

The lesson wasn't that dentistry failed her. The lesson was that timing matters. Her system needed to become structurally coherent enough to tolerate a meaningful dental change without interpreting it as threat.

When she eventually worked with an orthodontist who approached her case differently—not by polishing the existing bite, but by rebuilding its architecture with the whole system in mind—she felt something she hadn't felt in a long time: certainty. Not hype. Not hope.

The sensation that her nervous system had finally stopped arguing with the input.

Kim teaches the third lesson:

When the bite is the biggest remaining driver, nothing else holds. But when the sequence is right, the system can integrate with a speed and clarity that makes the earlier struggle look almost unfair.

WHY "DENTISTRY FIRST" IS RARELY THE BEST STRATEGY

Correcting the bite before correcting the base is like tuning a violin during an earthquake. If the pelvis is torsioned, if the rib cage is rotating around it, if the CCJ is working overtime to keep the eyes level, and if the breathing strategy is already defensive, the bite is trying to stabilize on a moving platform.

That's why so many well-intended dental interventions seem to "fail": the nervous system can't stabilize around a structure it perceives as unclear, unsafe, or inconsistent.

This is also why, in a Teeth-to-Toes model, we often can't evaluate the bite cleanly until the system beneath it is coherent enough to tell the truth. When the lower body and the orientation system are noisy, the bite you see may not be the bite that matters.

It may be a temporary survival arrangement—an adaptive best guess created by a nervous system doing its job.

That doesn't make dentistry less important. It makes dentistry more precise.

And it makes timing non-negotiable.

THE PRECISION OF MICRONS

Once you understand what the bite truly is—a sensory reference system, not just tooth contact—the need for precision stops being surprising.

In a system where distress can be triggered by microns and millimetres, "almost right" may not be right enough. A correction delivered at the wrong moment may not integrate. And a bite prescription that ignores the whole-body context can destabilize the very thing it's trying to help.

When the sequence is right and the prescription is right, patients describe something in plain language that clinicians recognize immediately:

The system stops defending. Breath drops. The jaw softens without being forced. The neck stops "working." The body feels more centered—not because we chased symmetry, but because we reduced confusion.

WHAT THIS CHAPTER IS ACTUALLY AN ARGUMENT FOR

This chapter isn't an argument for dentistry-first, and it isn't an argument for dentistry-last.

It's a call to recognize that the bite can be an essential contributor to Teeth-to-Toes physiology—and that ignoring it carries real risk in complex cases.

It's also an argument for sequencing: outcomes often depend as much on when an intervention takes place as on what is done. For many clinicians, that feels radical not because it's complicated, but because it forces humility. It forces us to admit that a good tool, used at the wrong time, can fail—or even backfire.

And finally, it's an argument for restraint: a bite often can't be evaluated cleanly until the system beneath it is coherent enough to tell the truth.

Raji shows what happens when the bite destabilizes the system early. Julie warns that the right idea delivered too soon can provoke a protective storm. Kim shows the payoff when the system is ready to integrate the final piece.

Taken together, these cases point to the safeguard that keeps any model—no matter how elegant—from becoming dogma:

Test. Intervene. Retest.

That is where we go next.

PART THREE

How To Apply It

ORDER, STRATEGY, AND DURABILITY

Understanding protection is not enough.

Identifying gateways is not enough.

Order determines outcome.

Sequence determines stability.

Maintenance determines longevity.

This section outlines how to apply the framework in practice—whether restoring your own body or guiding someone else through the process.

CHAPTER 10

Common Misconceptions

WHAT MODERN REHAB GETS WRONG (AND WHY)

FOUR CONCEPTUAL ERRORS THAT KEEP GOOD PEOPLE STUCK

By the time a complex patient finds their way into a Teeth-to-Toes conversation, they've often accumulated something more damaging than pathology: competing explanations. Smart, conscientious clinicians can look at the same person and tell four different stories—each coherent within its own discipline—while the patient becomes the unwilling project manager of an argument nobody is having out loud.

This chapter exists to prevent the most predictable failure that follows any powerful model: turning it into an ideology. Teeth-to-Toes isn't a belief system. It's a way of thinking that stays honest through a single, unfashionable standard:

Test. Intervene. Retest.

If an explanation is real, it should help predict outcomes. If it predicts outcomes, it should survive contact with a body—quickly, measurably, and repeatedly. If it can't be tested, it eventually becomes a story people defend instead of a model that helps people heal.

With that standard in mind, here are four conceptual errors that most reliably keep good clinicians—and their patients—stuck.

MISCONCEPTION 1: THE PROBLEM IS EITHER "STRUCTURAL" OR "SENSITIZATION"

This is the most damaging misconception because it forces a false choice at the very beginning of reasoning. Either the patient is "mechanical," or they're "central." Either the tissues are the problem, or the nervous system is. Either we chase anatomy, or we chase psychology. That binary can sound sophisticated. It isn't. It's a shortcut disguised as wisdom.

Clinical reality: pain is an output—an intelligent, protective decision made by a nervous system assessing threat in real time. That decision draws from multiple inputs: prior injury history, sleep and stress physiology, immune activation, movement options, tissue capacity, autonomic tone, and yes—mechanical load, asymmetry, and orientation.

This is where the word *sensitization* needs a plain-English translation. Sensitization doesn't mean pain is imagined, exaggerated, or "all in your head." It means the system's alarm threshold has dropped. When the nervous system has been managing threat and load long enough, it becomes easier to trigger protective output—more volume for the same input, less tolerance before the system says enough.

In that state, a mechanically unclear body doesn't just hurt more easily; it often recovers more slowly, tolerates change less well, and can flare in ways that confuse both patient and practitioner.

Modern pain science didn't eliminate biomechanics. It expanded the model. The nervous system doesn't float above structure; it lives inside it. A nervous system can be sensitized and mechanically overloaded at the same time—and those states often reinforce each other: mechanical confusion drives protection, and chronic protection lowers threshold.

What this looks like in clinic is painfully familiar. A patient is told, with good intent, "This is sensitization," and is encouraged to relax, reframe, and gradually expose themselves to movement. They try. They work hard. They even feel empowered—until every attempt to build activity collapses into the same pattern: guarding, breath tightening, jaw clenching, sleep disruption, and a flare that seems to arrive "for no reason."

Nothing is wrong with the concept. What's missing is an honest mechanical audit. If the pelvis is torsioned, the rib cage is braced, or the head is living in an orientation strategy, then the system is being asked to downshift while still managing a crooked reference point. In those cases, reassurance becomes a noble idea with an incomplete plan.

Practical takeaway: stop asking, "Is it mechanical or nervous system?" Ask: **Which inputs are keeping this system in protection—and which ones can we change first?** That question keeps you out of ideology and inside clinical work.

MISCONCEPTION 2: IF IMAGING IS "MILD," THE PROBLEM CAN'T BE SERIOUS

This misconception is subtle because it often comes wrapped in reassurance—and reassurance matters. The problem isn't the intent. The problem is the conclusion: if imaging doesn't look dramatic, then the symptoms must be disproportionate, exaggerated, or purely psychological.

That framing injures people twice: first by leaving the primary driver unaddressed, and second by making them doubt their own experience.

Clinical reality: imaging is excellent at many things. It is also famously limited at explaining lived physiology in complex, load-sensitive cases. A system can be structurally "fine" on paper and still be functionally expensive to operate. Conversely, imaging can look frightening and be clinically quiet. Neither outcome is rare.

Teeth-to-Toes doesn't argue against imaging. It argues against using imaging as a substitute for reasoning. The nervous system organizes around function—orientation, load transfer, stability, breath behavior, threat level—not around radiology reports.

A patient has a scan showing "mild degeneration," is told nothing serious is wrong, and is sent away with generic advice. Months later they return worse—not because degeneration suddenly accelerated, but because the driver was never what was revealed by the scan. The driver was load: a pelvis that can't distribute force cleanly, a bite that behaves like a vise, a neck that stays on vigilance to keep the eyes level, and a diaphragm that has been bracing like armor for years.

When you change that driver—even slightly—something diagnostic often happens. The person stands differently. Breath drops. Gait smooths. Facial tone changes. The system looks less defended. That isn't placebo. That's the nervous system responding to reduced demand.

Practical takeaway: use imaging to rule out what must be ruled out. Then return to the work that predicts outcomes: function, response, and durability. If a change lowers load, the system should show it.

MISCONCEPTION 3: THE LOUDEST SYMPTOM IS THE PRIMARY PROBLEM

This is the trap that catches even excellent clinicians, because it's human nature to treat what is shouting. The jaw is screaming, so we chase the jaw. The low back is raging, so we chase the low back. The neck feels "unstable," so we chase the neck.

Sometimes that is correct. Often it is incomplete.

Clinical reality: the body is not obligated to hurt where it is most distorted, and it is not obligated to signal where the primary driver lives. Pain is not a GPS coordinate. It is a protective message. In a load-managed system, symptoms often show up where compensation is failing—not where the original distortion began.

This is why Teeth-to-Toes keeps returning to the same question: **What is placing the greatest load on this nervous system right now?** Not what hurts the most. Not what looks most dramatic. Not what a single discipline is trained to prioritize.

What this looks like in clinic can be maddening until the pattern clicks. A patient arrives for "TMJ dysfunction," and everyone's eyes go to the jaw—yet the jaw is behaving like a stabilizer because the rib cage is locked and the head is living forward of the body's midline.

Or a patient arrives for "low back pain," and every intervention is local—until someone checks the pelvis and finds a torsion pattern that has been steering the entire chain. When the primary driver is reduced, the loud symptom often changes first—not because it was the cause, but because it was the cost.

Practical takeaway: the symptom is the flare. The driver is the fuel. Treating the flare can be compassionate and necessary, but recovery depends on finding—and reducing—the fuel.

MISCONCEPTION 4: SEQUENCE IS OPTIONAL—IF THE PARTS ARE TRUE, THE ORDER SHOULDN'T MATTER

This is the misconception that keeps experienced clinicians humble, because they usually learn it only after watching "good work" fail to hold. The intervention is correct. The reasoning is solid. The provider is skilled. The patient improves—then collapses back to baseline, or flares, or becomes "mysterious."

At that point, the profession often defaults to personality explanations: compliance, motivation, fear, inconsistency. Sometimes those factors matter. Often, something simpler is true.

Clinical reality: outcomes can depend as much on *when* an intervention takes place as on *what* you did. That can feel radical, because it challenges the comforting fantasy that a good tool should work whenever it is applied.

But the nervous system is state-dependent. Timing and tolerance are not footnotes; they are governing variables. A system with low reserve cannot integrate big changes cleanly. A system still compensating for a crooked foundation may reject an upstream correction that would have worked beautifully later. A system already in vigilance may treat the right input as just one more demand.

This is not mysticism. It's dosage.

What this looks like in clinic is a familiar heartbreak. A patient receives a precise intervention—manual, dental, upper cervical, corrective exercise—and improves sharply. Then their body "doesn't hold it."

In a Teeth-to-Toes frame, the first question isn't "What went wrong?" It's **"What was still forcing this system to protect?"** If the pelvis is still distorted, the CCJ may not stabilize. If the control tower is still noisy, pelvic work may not persist. If breath remains defensive, the system may stay in threat even with better geometry.

If the bite is evaluated before the rest of the system is coherent enough to tell the truth, the plan can be technically accurate and functionally destabilizing.

Practical takeaway: when a good intervention doesn't hold, don't assume failure. Assume sequence is still being discovered. Then test again.

THE FILTER THAT KEEPS YOU OUT OF IDEOLOGY

These misconceptions persist because each one contains a half-truth—and half-truths are persuasive.

The antidote is not a new belief. It's a standard.

Test a meaningful function. Apply a targeted input. Retest immediately. Then monitor durability. Keep what improves the whole-body result. Discard what doesn't—even if it is popular, familiar, or flattering to your discipline.

That isn't cynicism. It's respect—for time, for hope, and for the nervous system's limited capacity.

But there's one more safeguard worth naming, because it prevents Teeth-to-Toes from becoming the very thing it warns against: a framework that people use to win arguments instead of help bodies.

The safeguard is humility with teeth.

If your favourite explanation can't predict a retest, it doesn't get to run the case.

If a patient improves in a way your model cannot explain, you don't get to dismiss it—you get to expand your thinking.

If an intervention helps but doesn't hold, you don't double down on force—you look for the next limiter.

And if the system flares when you "should" be progressing, you don't blame the patient's character. You reassess the state of the nervous system and the cost of the demand you just applied.

That is how good clinicians stay honest.

BRIDGE TO CHAPTER ELEVEN — THE SEQUENCE

Now that we've cleared the conceptual fog, we can do what most books avoid: stop describing the problem and begin describing a usable strategy.

The next chapter is where Teeth-to-Toes becomes operational.

The Sequence is not a rigid algorithm, and it is not a turf war disguised as a framework. It is a way of deciding what the body can tolerate, what it is currently using as a stabilizer, and what must be addressed first if we want changes to hold.

Order matters. Dose matters. Durability matters.

And once you understand why, the hardest cases stop feeling mysterious. They start behaving like systems.

That is where we go next.

CHAPTER 11

The Sequence

WHY ORDER DETERMINES OUTCOME

Part II gave you the gateways—the pelvis, the CCJ, the breath, and the bite—and showed how an overwhelmed nervous system can recruit any of them as a stabilizer when load climbs and orientation becomes uncertain. Chapter Ten cleared away the conceptual fog that keeps good people debating what's true instead of testing what holds.

Now we pivot from understanding to application—from why complex cases stall to how they begin moving again.

There is a moment in almost every durable recovery when the nervous system stops resisting and allows a correction to take root. Clinicians recognize it. Patients feel it. The body expresses it. Sometimes it arrives like a lightning strike; sometimes it unfolds like a thaw. Either way, it is not magic. It is neurological acceptance—the point at which the system recognizes that the primary load it has been fighting has finally dropped far enough to be safe.

When that happens, intelligent biology does what intelligent systems always do: it reallocates resources. Bracing softens. Balance improves. Guarding decreases. Movement options expand. Vigilance quiets. Healing becomes metabolically affordable again.

That shift is not always instant. Rachel's recovery unfolded more like a sunrise than a switch. Her pelvis straightened within minutes. Her hip pain quieted that day. But the deeper change—the sense that her system trusted the new organization—took weeks. Many Teeth-to-Toes recoveries take longer still, often months and sometimes years, because the bucket has been full for so long and load-bearing structures have been compensating for decades.

And yet the architecture of durable outcomes is remarkably consistent:

Reduce the primary driver.

Stabilize what changed.

Rebuild the capacity to stay there.

In hypermobile systems, that middle step is decisive. When passive connective tissue provides less structural restraint, the nervous system must generate more active stability to feel safe. If stabilization is rushed or skipped, the system often reverts—not because the correction was wrong, but because the new geometry never became trustworthy enough to hold.

If you remember only one line from this chapter, make it this:

Sequence determines success—not because the body is fragile, but because the body is organized. And organization has rules.

PRIMARY DRIVERS ARE INDIVIDUAL AND TIME-DEPENDENT

One of the most persistent errors in rehabilitation is the belief that there must be a single structure that is always primary.

There isn't.

But there is always something that is primary.

In this framework, *primary* does not mean "the only thing that matters." It means the current dominant driver—the structure or system placing the greatest organizing demand on the nervous system right now. The one everything else is adapting around. The one the body is protecting at the highest cost.

Ken's case revealed a pelvis so distorted that nothing upstream could function cleanly until it was corrected. Once the foundation straightened, decades of knee pain vanished—not because the knee was treated, but because the system no longer needed to protect it.

Sean's case showed the opposite. His cranio-cervical junction was the dominant driver, destabilizing orientation and pushing his nervous system into a survival-grade state. Without upper cervical care, no amount of exercise, manual therapy, or postural coaching would have held, because the control tower could not tolerate the demand.

Kim's case demonstrated a third pattern. Her pelvis and CCJ required correction first, but the final barrier lived in the bite. Only when dental intervention was delivered at the right moment did her system finally release its grip and reorganize.

Each discipline mattered most—at different moments, for different bodies.

That insight prevents needless turf wars. The entry point is not universal. It is earned through assessment.

Primary does not mean permanent.

Primary means first—for this person, at this time.

Two people can share similar symptoms and require radically different starting points—not because anyone is wrong, but because their nervous systems are protecting against different drivers.

WHAT SEQUENCE LOOKS LIKE IN REAL LIFE

Sequence is not a rigid protocol. It is not Step 1, Step 2, Step 3 applied mechanically to everyone. Complex systems do not behave that way.

Sequence is closer to navigation than to a recipe. You begin by locating yourself. Then you choose the first move that reduces risk, improves orientation, and gives the system a better chance of holding the next change.

Clinically, that means identifying the dominant driver, reducing it, observing the response, and reassessing what is now visible—because you can only see the next problem clearly once the primary one is quiet enough to stop distorting everything downstream.

People can spend years doing the "right things" in the wrong order and feel as though their body is sabotaging them. It is not sabotage. It is hierarchy. The nervous system will protect the most urgent threat first and will gladly sacrifice comfort elsewhere if that is what survival-grade organization requires.

CASE ANCHOR: THE VILLAGE SQUAT — WHEN THE BODY TELLS THE TRUTH

Across disciplines, we all return to the same question at key moments: what does the body look like when we let it stand and organize itself without coaching?

Relaxed stance is one of the simplest ways to see whether the system is quieter, more coherent, and less defended than it was a few minutes ago. The Village Squat belongs in that same category of high-signal tools.

It is a corrective exercise, yes—but like the best correctives, it can also reveal compensation patterns in the major weightbearing joints and spine. In the right context, it becomes a live demonstration of the clinical standard that keeps this model honest:

Test something meaningful.

Apply one specific input.

Retest immediately.

A squat is honest. It exposes limits the body has been negotiating quietly: ankle motion, knee tracking, hip depth, pelvic symmetry, spinal strategy, and—most importantly—how all those pieces cooperate under gravity.

Before intervention, the cost is often visible without imaging. The torso may list subtly to one side. The low back may appear rigid. One hip may sit in quiet rotation. The knees may not track symmetrically. The feet may angle outward as if straight ahead is unavailable. Breathing often stays high and shallow—not necessarily from anxiety, but because bracing has become the default.

The overall impression is diagnostic: the system is working hard just to tolerate standing. Standing should not feel like endurance work.

Then you give the system one precise stimulus. Sometimes that stimulus is a squat-pattern hold—feet parallel, knees wide, the posture of a frog—held briefly and supported if necessary. Nothing heroic. Nothing dramatic. Just enough input for the nervous system to decide whether it is safe to reorganize.

Most beginners require a supported version first—sometimes for weeks—until the nervous system trusts the shape enough to release bracing. Support lowers threat. Lower threat reveals truth.

Then you retest. If the chosen stimulus reduced meaningful load—especially if it touched the primary driver—the body often looks different within minutes. The torso lists less. The low back stops gripping. The pelvis appears straighter. Hip rotation softens. Breath drops. The whole system looks quieter.

Occasionally, the position that looked nearly impossible moments earlier becomes tolerable, even effortless—not because the person "opened up," and not because they "got stronger," but because the nervous system decided it was safe enough to stop protecting.

That is neurological acceptance in miniature.

TWO SIMPLE TESTS THAT CLARIFY SEQUENCE

These tests do not replace expert care, and they are not magic tricks. They simply allow the body to declare, in real time, whether an upstream input is organizing the system.

The Cervical Syndrome Test – A Window into CCJ Load

With the person lying on their back and legs extended, the clinician aligns the heels to observe subtle differences in length. The person then slowly turns the head left and returns to center, then right and returns.

In some cases, turning the head one direction makes one leg appear to shorten slightly; turning the other direction restores symmetry.

This is not diagnosing pathology. It is revealing organization. A change in head position alters tone below. The nervous system is spending resources protecting orientation.

When that pattern is clear sequence may change. Addressing the control tower early may provide more durability than continuing to work downstream while orientation remains unstable.

The Teeth-to-Toes Test — Does Bite Stability Change Global Organization?

Standing, the person lifts one knee and extends the same-side arm. Gentle downward pressure is applied to the arm as the person resists. You observe steadiness and ease.

Then you introduce temporary bite contact—something as simple as a small object placed lightly between the teeth—and repeat the test.

If stability and strength expression improve meaningfully, the bite is functioning as an upstream organizing input.

This does not prove dentistry first. It reveals whether dentistry is likely to matter in that person's sequence.

A CLEAR, TESTABLE ARCHITECTURE

Although the entry point varies, durable recoveries tend to follow a recognizable structure.

Phase One: Corrective — Reduce the Primary Driver

This phase is not strengthening. It is not performance. It is identifying and reducing the dominant driver—the factor placing the greatest load on the system at that moment.

When the primary driver is reduced, feedback is often immediate: breath slows, facial tone changes, gait looks less guarded, a headache fades, a jaw unclenches.

The work is iterative: correct, reassess, refine—not until perfection, but until the nervous system signals that the major load has dropped beneath its protection threshold.

Remove load before adding demand.

Phase Two: Stabilization — Teach the Body Its New Reality

Once load is reduced, the system must learn to hold the change. This phase is especially critical in hypermobile systems, where passive restraint is limited and active stability must increase.

Corrective exercise becomes a teaching tool, not a forcing tool. The aim is to reinforce new geometry so the nervous system stops borrowing stability from the jaw, ribs, neck, or low back.

Patients often describe this phase not as "stronger," but as "stable." Stability is one of the clearest signs that protection is giving way to efficiency.

Phase Three: Maintenance — Preserve Margin

The final phase is not an endpoint but a strategy. Small routines, applied intelligently, help preserve pelvic neutrality, diaphragmatic mobility, CCJ support, and bite stability.

Life remains demanding. Maintenance preserves margin so flare-ups become shorter, rarer, and less frightening.

WHY ORDER IS (ALMOST) EVERYTHING

A difficult truth becomes easier to accept once sequence is understood: the wrong intervention at the wrong time is not neutral. It can be destabilizing.

Address the bite before the pelvis is stable and the orthotic may fail—not because dentistry is flawed, but because the floor is moving. Push strengthening before reducing load and the nervous system may interpret effort as threat. Correct the pelvis while the CCJ is dominating orientation and the change may not hold.

Two clinicians can use the same tool with opposite outcomes. The tool is not the determining factor. The timing is.

Rachel's case made this clear. Skilled providers worked carefully within their domains, yet no one asked the decisive question: what is the primary driver for her, right now?

Her pelvis had never been meaningfully assessed for asymmetry. Once corrected, everything downstream reorganized—not because she believed in the correction, but because her nervous system finally had permission to stop protecting.

That is neurological acceptance in action.

BRIDGE TO THE ROADMAP

Sequence is the principle: order matters, timing matters, and the nervous system's tolerance is the limiting variable in complex cases.

The next chapter translates that principle into a practical Roadmap—how to identify the entry point, how to test the system without provoking it, and how to progress change in a way that holds.

That is where we go next.

CHAPTER 12

The Roadmap

FROM CORRECTION TO CAPACITY

By the time you reach this chapter, you've already absorbed the central lesson of *The Sequence*: complex pain rarely resolves because the right tool was finally found. It resolves when the right driver is reduced—at the right time, in the right order, and at a dose the nervous system can tolerate.

That chapter gave us the rule of the road: outcomes depend on priority, timing, and tolerance—not ideology, tradition, or whichever discipline speaks the loudest. But insight alone doesn't change outcomes. At some point, every patient—and every clinician—still asks the same question:

What do we do next?

This chapter is the answer to that question. Not as a protocol. Not as a recipe. As a map.

A map doesn't guarantee an easy hike. It simply keeps you from mistaking the swamp for the path.

WHAT THE ROADMAP IS REALLY TRACKING

Most people assume recovery is about fixing a structure: a disc, a joint, a muscle, a pattern. In a Teeth-to-Toes frame, recovery is usually about something more governing:

The moment the nervous system stops spending its budget on protection and starts spending it on reorganization.

That moment can feel dramatic—like a light turning on. More often it feels like weather changing: a thaw, a clearing, a subtle shift where the body begins behaving as though it is no longer bracing against itself. It isn't magic, and it isn't mindset.

It is what happens when load drops beneath a threshold the system can finally afford.

This is why the Roadmap exists: to help you find that threshold without accidentally adding threat in the name of help.

A QUICK CASE OVERLAY: KIM, AS NAVIGATION—NOT A STORY

Kim belongs here for one reason only: she shows what the Roadmap is doing in real time.

As her system became more coherent—first in her foundation, then in her orientation—the body didn't simply improve.

It revealed.

The quieter she became, the clearer the remaining driver became. The bite emerged not as the beginning of her story, but as what became visible once earlier drivers stopped dominating the screen.

Nothing prior was wasted. Each step reduced enough noise for the next truth to appear.

That's the Roadmap in its simplest form: not chasing symptoms, but steadily reducing the cost of being upright until the system stops arguing with the input.

THE ROADMAP IN ONE SENTENCE

Reduce the primary driver, stabilize what changed, and build the capacity to keep it.

Every durable recovery—no matter how complex—tends to follow that architecture. The entry point varies. The sequence is discovered. But the structure of progress repeats.

BEFORE PHASES: ASSESSMENT IS STATE-DEPENDENT

One of the most common reasons clinicians miss the primary driver is that they only ever look at the body in one condition.

The nervous system does not behave the same way under full demand as it does when demand is removed. If you don't account for that, you can end up treating the **shape** of compensation instead of the **source** of it.

- **Supine** often shows what the body does when it feels safer. Gravity stops interrogating the frame, tone can drop, bracing can soften, and some asymmetries reduce—not because the case is solved, but because the nervous system is no longer forced to hold the same strategy.
- **Standing** shows what the body does when it must perform. Gravity asks its question again, the righting reflex comes online, and whatever the nervous system has been doing to keep the head level and the airway stable becomes more obvious.

Neither state is "better." Each is a different truth.

The Roadmap is built on using both.

PHASE ONE: THE CORRECTIVE PHASE

Draining the Bucket—One Driver at a Time

The corrective phase is not strengthening, activation, or posture drills. It is the careful, sometimes stubborn work of identifying and reducing the **primary driver**: the structure or system placing the greatest organizing demand on the nervous system *right now*.

Sometimes that driver is pelvic torsion—the base is crooked, and everything above it is negotiating. Sometimes it is CCJ disorganization—the compass is noisy, and the whole body tightens to protect orientation. Sometimes it is breath and airway strategy—the system cannot downshift because air doesn't feel secure. Sometimes it is the bite—sensory input at the jaw is unclear enough that clenching becomes a stabilizer and never fully lets go.

Often more than one gateway matters. But in most cases, one gateway is costing the system the most **today**.

That is what *primary* means here.

And primary does not mean permanent. Primary means first—for this person, at this time.

What "success" looks like in Phase One

People expect success to look like less pain. Sometimes it does.

But the more reliable early sign is that the system becomes less defended.

Breath drops without coaching. Facial tone changes. Gait becomes quieter. Jaw tension eases between words. The neck stops "working" so hard just to exist. The body looks less like it is bracing against gravity and more like it is cooperating with it.

Those are not vague wellness markers. They are output changes—signs that load just fell beneath a threshold the nervous system can tolerate.

Why this phase is iterative by design

Phase One isn't where you "do the program." It's where you test the model.

You correct, reassess, correct again, and reassess again—not until everything is perfect, but until the nervous system signals, in its own language:

This is the doorway.

For some people, that doorway appears quickly. For others, it takes months. For the most complex cases, it can take longer.

The principle doesn't change:

Remove load before you add demand.

PHASE TWO: THE STABILIZATION PHASE

Teaching the Body Its New Reality

If Phase One lowers the cost of being upright, Phase Two teaches the nervous system to trust the new geometry.

This is where many well-intended plans quietly fail. People improve, then lose it, and the experience gets named as a flare, a slip, or proof that it "didn't hold."

Often nothing mysterious happened.

The system simply never developed enough stability to stop protecting.

This is especially decisive in hypermobile bodies, where passive connective tissue provides less restraint. In those systems, the nervous system must generate more active stability to feel safe. If stabilization is rushed or skipped, the system reverts—not because the correction was wrong, but because the new position never became trustworthy enough to keep.

Stabilization is not forcing

Corrective exercise is often misunderstood here, because the goal is rarely "strengthening weak muscles" in isolation.

In chronic cases, weakness is frequently a symptom of disorganization. A braced system can feel weak because it cannot distribute load efficiently, so it fatigues, shakes, and fails under demand—not due to insufficient horsepower, but because the nervous system doesn't trust the geometry it's operating inside.

Stabilization is neurological education: repeated, tolerable exposures to a cleaner alignment so the system stops borrowing stability from the jaw, the neck, the ribs, or the low back.

Patients often describe this phase with a word that matters:

"I don't feel stronger. I feel... **stable**."

That word is the felt experience of neurological acceptance.

The hidden danger of too much, too soon

In stabilization, dosage is everything.

Too much too soon and the nervous system reads the new demand as threat, returning to protection.

Too little for too long and the new position never becomes default.

So Phase Two is paced, monitored, and retested—not because the patient is fragile, but because the nervous system is precise.

PHASE THREE: THE MAINTENANCE PHASE

Resilience as a Learned State

Maintenance is not a finish line. It is what prevents quiet regression.

It's where the Minimum Effective Dose becomes a lifelong strategy: small, intelligent routines that keep the pelvis neutral, rib mechanics mobile, the diaphragm less guarded, the CCJ less burdened, and the bite less recruited as a stabilizer.

Gravity never retires. Stress doesn't stop applying load. Life will always test the structure.

Maintenance is how you stop making the nervous system relearn the same lesson every year.

This is also where recovery stops being a concept and becomes a lived state.

Sleep isn't a lifestyle cliché; it's a load-management tool. Breath isn't a trend; it's a dashboard. Pacing isn't weakness; it's strategy. Reserve isn't luck; it's built.

In Maintenance, flare-ups may still happen, but they become shorter, rarer, and less frightening—not because life becomes perfect, but because the system has margin again.

WHY THE ROADMAP WORKS

The Four Gateways are not separate systems. They are a conversation.

A crooked pelvis forces compensation upward. A noisy CCJ drives vigilance downward. A defensive breath keeps threat online. An unclear bite can destabilize orientation in microns.

The Roadmap works because it doesn't worship any one gateway. It simply asks—repeatedly—what is costing this system the most right now, and then does something simple but rare in modern care:

Test. Intervene. Retest.

Keep what lowers the whole-body cost of being upright.

WHEN THE ROADMAP FAILS

It's Usually Not Because the Tool Was Wrong

When a good intervention doesn't hold, the temptation is to call it failure—or to blame the patient with words like compliance, fear, inconsistency, or motivation.

Sometimes those variables matter.

Often something simpler is true:

The sequence is still being discovered.

A bite change can be correct and still destabilizing if the base is moving. Pelvic correction can be real and still temporary if orientation remains noisy. Breathwork can be helpful and still backfire if the rib cage can't move and the system interprets the demand as threat. Upper cervical correction can be precise and still fail to hold if the bite is feeding distortion back into the head–neck system.

The Roadmap doesn't judge those outcomes.

It reads them.

The body is not arguing with you.

It is informing you.

BRIDGE TO THE NEXT CHAPTER

The Roadmap is not a promise of speed. It is a promise of honesty.

It prevents the most expensive kind of failure: doing good work in the wrong order, then mistaking the nervous system's protective response for mystery—or moral weakness.

Once you understand this, the hardest cases stop feeling haunted. They start behaving like systems.

Not simple systems, but intelligible ones—systems with priorities, thresholds, and rules.

The next chapter moves from map to daily life: how to protect hard-won gains, keep load from quietly rebuilding, and live inside a body with enough reserve to heal.

That is where we go next.

CHAPTER 13

Maintenance

KEEPING THE BUCKET FROM FILLING AGAIN

When the Body Stops Borrowing From Tomorrow

People don't come to a book like this because they want a new hobby. They come because they want their life back.

By the time someone reaches Maintenance, they've already endured the part of recovery that feels like work: the experiments, the false starts, the flare-ups that seemed to erase progress overnight, and the constant question of whether the body is improving—or simply behaving for a day. They've learned what it means to be load-sensitive. They've learned, too, that the nervous system doesn't accept change because you understand it; it accepts change when the inputs become coherent enough—and safe enough—to hold.

Maintenance is what you do once the system has stopped fighting you. Not because you've finished, but because you've finally earned a baseline worth protecting.

Maintenance Is Not an Admission of Fragility

The word *maintenance* can trigger a reflex. Either: *So I'll have to do this forever?* Or: *If I have to maintain it, it wasn't real.*

Both reactions come from the same misunderstanding: that recovery should mean you never have to think about your body again.

That's not how biology works. You don't graduate from gravity. You don't outgrow stress. Sleep debt still counts. Travel still counts. Work posture still counts. Old injuries still count. A difficult season of life can refill the bucket without a dramatic event—simply by asking more than your reserve can afford.

Maintenance isn't a concession. It's how you protect capacity, so the system doesn't quietly run out of margin and then call it an injury.

Maintenance Is Biological Hygiene

Most people understand dental care intuitively. You don't visit a dentist because you're weak, and you don't brush and floss because you're broken. You do it because plaque forms, because bacteria exist, and because biology is dynamic. Teeth live in a system that never stops being used.

Biomechanical and neuromuscular health is no different. Gravity never retires. Stress never disappears. Load accumulates quietly. Life keeps happening.

If you had a cavity filled and then stopped brushing, nobody would blame the dentist when decay returned. They'd recognize something simpler: hygiene stopped. The same logic applies here. Corrective care restores organization. Maintenance preserves it.

And just like dental hygiene, maintenance doesn't require obsession—it requires consistency plus reassessment. Brushing your teeth doesn't eliminate the need for check-ups; it keeps you stable between them, and it helps you catch small drift before it gets expensive. The same is true here: self-care protects the gains you earned, and periodic reassessment protects you from guessing when the pattern changes.

The Real Goal of Maintenance

The goal isn't perfect posture. It's a body that stays organized without having to borrow from emergency strategies—jaw clenching, rib bracing, neck vigilance, pelvic torsion—just to get through a normal day.

In Maintenance, you're protecting four things:

- **Clarity** — clean reference points the nervous system can trust.
- **Capacity** — enough reserve that normal life doesn't trigger protection.
- **Durability** — changes that hold under real-world demand, not just in clinic.
- **Early detection** — noticing drift before it becomes suffering.

That's the quiet genius of Maintenance: it shifts you from reactive care to preemptive care, without turning your life into therapy.

Minimum Effective Dose

Maintenance fails when effort gets misunderstood. Some people overdo it, turning good habits into a new form of load. Others do nothing until the system forces them back into crisis mode.

The antidote is a principle every experienced clinician eventually learns, and every patient eventually appreciates:

Minimum Effective Dose — the smallest amount of intelligent input that keeps the system stable.

It's extremely valuable to know what your body requires to maintain stability, mobility, and comfort. Everyone is different. What is sufficient and appropriate for you may be far too aggressive for your neighbor. The goal here isn't maximal effort; it's sustainable organization—the kind your nervous system can afford on real days, not just good ones.

What You Maintain Is Not "The Exercises"

Many people make Maintenance strangely moral. They treat a routine as if it proves virtue—*I did my stretches; I'm a good person*—or they treat missing a day as failure—*I skipped it; I'm back at square one.*

Maintenance isn't about loyalty to a routine. It's about maintaining the state that routine creates.

In Teeth-to-Toes terms, you're protecting the stability of the Four Gateways:

- a pelvis neutral enough for efficient force transfer
- a CCJ quiet enough that orientation doesn't trigger vigilance
- breath low enough that the system can downshift and recover
- a bite coherent enough that the jaw doesn't become a splint

If those are holding, the details of how you maintain them can evolve.

The Maintenance Dashboard

People ask, *How will I know I'm slipping?*

You won't always feel pain first. Often the earliest signs are subtler—and more useful—because they arrive before the storm:

- breath rising into the chest
- the jaw returning during focus, driving, stress, or sleep
- standing becoming work again, as if you can't quite settle
- recovery thinning; sleep becoming lighter
- asymmetry creeping back in—a hip that grips, a hamstring that tugs, a shoulder that lives higher

None of that means you're broken again.

It means the bucket is filling.

And in Maintenance, you respond early—while the correction is still cheap.

Response and a Few Tools Worth Naming

Response means two things, and both are done early—calmly, not heroically.

First, you return to the self-care that already proved itself during your corrective phase: the handful of inputs that reliably improve your coherence, the few go-to correctives that consistently move the needle for you.

Second, you seek reassessment whether the pattern seems to resolve or not, because the nervous system is communicating something simple and urgent: it can't afford to wait. In that moment, you don't yet know whether what you're feeling is incidental or significant, and guessing is how small drift becomes a bigger problem.

Most maintenance tools are personal, earned through trial, retest, and time. But a few show up so often in load-sensitive bodies that they deserve special mention.

Gentle diaphragmatic breathing is close to universal—not as a performance drill and not as a fix, but as a way of lowering the cost of being you. And when the system needs something more structured, the strategies you learned earlier—**Box Breathing** and **4/7/8**—act like a reliable downshift lever: something you can reach for early, before vigilance hardens into a full-body storm. They don't force calm. They invite it, rhythmically, in a language the nervous system understands.

A squat-pattern exercise belongs on the same short list. It's one of the most efficient ways to keep the lower body honest—to maintain usable symmetry, mobility, and, when appropriate, strength—and it tends to reveal drift early, while the correction is still cheap.

And if your first thought is, *My back is too sore for that*, or *My knee won't bend that far*, or *That lights up my hip*—good. That's not failure; that's information. In almost every case, there's a modified version that meets your nervous system where it is: supine, wall-assisted, supported, or simply shallower—something that preserves the underlying shape without provoking protection.

Don't guess. Consult the expert on your team, and choose the version your body can actually accept.

One boundary protects all of this: individual differences aren't a footnote—they're the whole game. You wouldn't experiment with your friend's prescription drugs; don't do the rehab equivalent. Copying someone else's miracle routine and expecting the same outcome isn't discipline—it's gambling. Maintenance isn't about doing more. It's about doing what's right for your system, at a dose it can actually afford, so organization stays sustainable and life stays livable.

When Maintenance Is Working

When maintenance is working, something subtle happens: you stop fearing flare-ups. Not because they never occur, but because when they do, they're shorter, quieter, more predictable, and less dramatic. You recognize the signs sooner. You intervene calmly. The body reorganizes. Life continues.

That's resilience—not the absence of stress, but the presence of margin.

The Difference Between Cure and Care

The fantasy most patients carry—understandably—is that recovery means never thinking about the problem again. That fantasy is reinforced by much of modern medicine: remove the lesion, repair the tissue, and move on.

But neuromechanical organization isn't a static repair. It's an ongoing relationship between gravity, load, and nervous system interpretation. The pelvis can drift. Breath can rise. The jaw can re-recruit. The CCJ can become vigilant again—not because the correction failed, but because life keeps applying load.

Maintenance isn't endless therapy.

It's ongoing care.

And the people who thrive long-term aren't the ones who do the most. They're the ones who notice early drift and respond before protection escalates.

That isn't fragility.

That's literacy.

The Final Principle

If there is one idea this entire book has been building toward, it is this:

The nervous system is not your enemy. It is your guardian.

When you reduce the load it must manage, it rewards you with stability. When you overload it, it protects you.

Maintenance is simply respecting that contract.

Just as brushing your teeth respects the biology of enamel and bacteria, neuromechanical hygiene respects the biology of gravity and load. It isn't dramatic. It isn't heroic.

It is intelligent.

And when practiced with humility, it allows something people often forget is possible:

A body that feels like home again.

BRIDGE TO THE EPILOGUE

You now understand how to stay well. The final question is deeper: what does it mean to live well once the body is no longer defending itself?

Because alignment is not only mechanical. It is behavioral. It is emotional. It is neurological. It is philosophical. A body in alignment is a nervous system in dialogue with itself—and a nervous system in dialogue with itself is a person free to live the life they were built for.

The Epilogue is where the Teeth-to-Toes journey stops being a rehabilitation model and becomes something more expansive: a way of being in the world.

Epilogue

THE WAY FORWARD

There is a moment in almost every patient's journey—quiet, almost unremarkable—when something extraordinary becomes undeniable.

They are no longer negotiating with their body. They are simply living.

It rarely arrives with fanfare. There is no swelling music, no triumphant announcement. It shows up in the smallest, most intimate ways: a morning when you step out of bed without bracing; a walk where breath feels unforced; a dinner where you are present instead of managing symptoms; a drive where the hip stays quiet; a night where the jaw rests instead of clenching into the dark.

And then, slowly and unmistakably, the thought lands:

This is what it feels like to be at ease inside myself.

This closing chapter is about that moment—and what it represents. Because Teeth-to-Toes is not merely "corrective exercise," or "atlas work," or "dental stabilization." It is a way of understanding the human body that restores dignity, restores agency, and restores the possibility of a future no longer dictated by symptoms.

Beneath all the science, all the stories, and all the structure of this book, one truth has been waiting in plain sight:

When the nervous system is no longer overwhelmed, the human being reappears.

THE GIFT OF CAPACITY

Most people do not arrive for care believing they are capable. By the time they walk into a clinic—any clinic—they often carry a private narrative: I'm fragile, my body betrayed me, this must be my new normal, maybe this is just who I am now.

Pain tells convincing stories.

But the nervous system has its own story, and it is far less fatalistic: capacity can be rebuilt. Load can be reduced. Threat can be drained. Organization can return.

And when it does, people rediscover abilities they thought were gone for good: the ability to work a full day without fearing the evening; to travel without strategizing every step; to play with their children without hesitation; to train again—stronger, smarter, more coherent. Most of all, the ability to trust their body again.

The greatest gift of this work isn't the disappearance of pain.

It's the return of capacity—that spacious, steady sense that there is finally enough bandwidth to live the life you choose.

THE END OF SELF-BLAME

Nearly every patient carries some version of guilt. Sometimes it's quiet, sometimes explicit: I should have been stronger, I should have stretched more, I should have known better.

But nothing in this book has ever been about blame. It has been about biology.

A tilted pelvis is not a character flaw. Forward head posture is not a moral failing. A dysfunctional bite is not a lack of discipline. A misaligned atlas is not a lifestyle choice. Trauma responses are not stubbornness. Compensation patterns are not carelessness. A full bucket is not weakness.

Every distortion your body adopted was an act of intelligence—an attempt to keep you upright, stable, and safe under conditions it could not solve cleanly.

Pain was not failure. Pain was communication.

When that truth lands—not intellectually, but viscerally—something profound happens:

People stop fighting themselves.

And that, more than any technique, is where healing begins.

WHAT WE FAIL TO SEE

By the time a system reaches collapse, the problem is rarely a lack of effort, intelligence, or care. It is almost always a limitation of framework.

Across this book you've met clinicians who were skilled, conscientious, and genuinely trying to help—yet still missed the driver that mattered most. Not because they were careless, but because the answer lived outside the borders of their training. The knee expert never thought to question the pelvis. The manual therapist never suspected a control-tower problem at the CCJ. The dental intervention arrived before the system was quiet enough to reveal what the bite was actually doing.

Each practitioner was working carefully within their domain. Each intervention made sense—until it didn't.

And when the body fails to respond, the most dangerous sentence in healthcare quietly enters the room:

We don't know.

As Dr. Javier Vasquez often reminds his colleagues, you can only treat what you can see—and you can only see what you were trained to see.

This is not a condemnation of modern care. It is simply the natural edge of any evolving model. The human body does not organize itself according to professional silos. It does not separate pelvis from spine, spine from breath, breath from bite, or structure from neurological load.

When care fragments the system, the truth fragments with it.

What changes outcomes is not necessarily a stronger intervention.

It is a wider lens.

When the lens expands, sequence becomes visible. When sequence becomes visible, the primary driver can finally be addressed. And when the primary driver drops, the nervous system stops fighting and starts reorganizing. That isn't ideology. It's physiology.

THE QUIET SECRET OF ALIGNMENT-CENTRIC CARE

Across these chapters we have talked about the pelvis, the CCJ, breath, airway, bite mechanics, autonomic load, proprioceptive clarity, and the Threat Bucket.

But the deeper thread running through all of it is simpler than it sounds:

What we are really restoring is coherence.

Mechanical coherence. Neurological coherence. Respiratory coherence. The kind of coherence that allows the system to stop improvising survival strategies and return to something far more efficient: organized function.

An aligned body is not just straighter; it is integrated. The pelvis informs the spine. The spine informs the ribs. The ribs inform the diaphragm. The diaphragm shapes breath. Breath shapes state. State shapes tone—everywhere.

No part functions alone. No part heals alone. No part fails alone.

We do not fix body parts.

We restore the conversation between them.

A NEW NORMAL

When the system begins to hold, something changes in the patient's language. Maintenance becomes less like a chore and more like hygiene—simple, intelligent, and protective. The correctives shrink not because the work is being neglected, but because the work is no longer fighting upstream. Breath becomes intuitive. Awareness replaces vigilance. Confidence replaces fear.

And patients often say something that reveals the deepest shift of all:

"I can feel when I'm drifting."

That sentence is not trivial. It means the person is no longer living at the mercy of flare-ups, mystery, or panic. The early signals are recognizable. The response is calmer. Course-correction happens sooner—before protection escalates.

Resilience is not the absence of stress.

It is the presence of margin.

It is adaptability returned.

THE REAL MEANING OF TEETH-TO-TOES

The name may sound structural. The method may sound mechanical.

But the outcome is profoundly human.

Teeth-to-Toes is not a promise of perfection. It is permission for physiology to do what it was designed to do once load becomes manageable and reference points become trustworthy.

When the body is organized, the nervous system can breathe.

When the nervous system can breathe, the human being can live.

Not dramatically. Not heroically.

Simply—cleanly—day after day.

Your symptoms never defined you.

Your capacity does.

THE PATH AHEAD

You now have the map. You've seen the principles. You've met the patients. You've watched the system reorganize—pelvis to cranium, airway to autonomic state, survival to coherence.

The only question left is what you will do with this understanding.

If you are a clinician: widen your lens. Collaborate boldly. Test everything. Follow the sequence your patient's body reveals—not the one you were trained to assume.

If you are a patient: ask better questions. Protect your progress. Refuse fragmented care as your default ever again.

And if you are simply someone searching for answers: let this be the beginning—not the end—of how you understand your body. Because change does not begin with systems. It begins with people. Which means it begins with you.

The Biomechanical Brain is not the closing of a story.

It is the opening of one.

And I'm grateful—deeply, sincerely—to have walked this landscape with you.

Geoff Dakin
Calgary, Alberta, Canada
November 27, 2025

About the Authors

Geoff Dakin, BPE, RMT, is the founder of Alignment First Inc. and the creator of the Alignment First Protocol, a corrective-exercise system used internationally to address chronic pain and postural dysfunction. Based in Calgary, Alberta, Canada, Geoff has devoted nearly four decades to clinical practice, working with everyday pain sufferers and elite athletes alike, including a tenure as a therapist for the Vancouver Canucks of the National Hockey League. He is the Amazon best-selling author of *The Body Mechanic's Handbook* and a published researcher.

His work is grounded in a deceptively simple principle: when alignment improves, neurological load decreases—and the body regains capacity. Increasingly, his clinical focus has centered on integrating corrective exercise with upper cervical care, dentistry, and airway science into a unified framework that respects the body as an interconnected system rather than a collection of parts.

Jeffrey N. Scholten, BSc, DC, practices at The Vital Posture Clinic in Calgary, Alberta, Canada, where he focuses on precise cranio-cervical junction procedures. He is recognized by the International Chiropractors Association Council on Upper Cervical Care as both a Diplomate and Fellow, and by the Canadian Academy of Pain Management as a Diplomate in Pain Management.

Dr. Scholten has spent decades refining his understanding of how subtle orientation changes at the upper cervical spine influence balance, postural tone, and whole-body neurological organization. His work is defined by precision and restraint—small, exacting corrections that allow system-wide recalibration. He is widely respected for his thoughtful, evidence-informed approach to complex neuromusculoskeletal cases.

Dr. Curtis Westersund, DDS, practices at Dentalife in Calgary, Alberta, Canada, where his clinical focus bridges general dentistry with temporomandibular dysfunction (TMD), airway health, and the neurological implications of occlusion. Through years of treating complex and often refractory cases, he has become a leading advocate for viewing the bite not merely as a mechanical interface, but as a powerful sensory input capable of shaping posture, breathing, and nervous system regulation.

His work emphasizes interdisciplinary collaboration and a deeper understanding of how millimeters in the mouth can translate into meaningful changes throughout the body. By integrating dentistry into a broader neuromechanical framework, Dr. Westersund helps patients move beyond symptom management toward durable systemic coherence.

Glossary

Some terms in this glossary describe anatomical structures; others describe functional states, organizing principles, or patterns of nervous-system behavior. Many refer less to isolated parts than to relationships between them.

ADAPTATION

The body's intelligent, energy-efficient response to everyday demand. Adaptation is quiet and largely invisible; it allows you to remain upright, balanced, and functional without conscious effort. It reflects a nervous system that perceives sufficient safety and capacity. Problems arise only when adaptation is exhausted and compensation replaces it.
See also: Compensation, Load.

AIRWAY STRAIN

A subtle but powerful source of systemic load. When the airway is narrow, unstable, or crowded, the nervous system reorganizes posture, rib mechanics, tongue position, and jaw tension to preserve airflow. Airway strain often influences alignment long before obvious symptoms appear.
See also: Breath Mechanics, Tongue Posture, Autonomic Load.

ALIGNMENT

Not a cosmetic ideal, but the structural condition that allows gravity to pass through the body with minimal friction. Alignment reduces neurological demand by making posture, movement, and breathing easier to sustain. When alignment deteriorates, the nervous system compensates—often silently—until symptoms emerge. Alignment is not the final goal; it is the gateway to neurological ease.

ATLAS (C1)

The top vertebra of the spine and one of the most neurologically consequential structures in the body. Subtle orientation changes here can influence balance, visual reference, airway behavior, and reflexive tone throughout the system. Its impact derives from sensory clarity rather than strength.
See also: CCJ, Upper Cervical Care.

AUTONOMIC NERVOUS SYSTEM (ANS)

The regulatory branch of the nervous system governing heart rate, digestion, breathing rhythm, and baseline muscle tone. It continuously evaluates threat and safety. When mechanical distortion or chronic stress increases load, the ANS may shift toward sympathetic dominance. Healing accelerates when the system perceives enough safety to downshift.
See also: Sympathetic Dominance, Neurological Acceptance.

AUTONOMIC LOAD

The cumulative physiological demand imposed by mechanical distortion, emotional stress, trauma history, inefficient breathing, poor sleep, and unresolved compensation. High autonomic load reduces adaptability and lowers the threshold for protective responses—even when tissue damage is absent.

BITE (OCCLUSION)

The meeting relationship of the teeth—and, more importantly, a sensory reference point informing jaw position, cranial mechanics, airway strategy, and upper cervical orientation. Small discrepancies in occlusion can produce significant neurological effects, particularly in systems already under load.
See also: TMJ, Micron.

BIOMECHANICAL COHERENCE

A state in which body segments cooperate rather than compete. Coherence feels like ease—fluid movement, stable posture, responsive balance, and unforced breathing. When coherence is lost, the nervous system must spend energy maintaining orientation rather than refining function.
See also: Alignment, Neurological Acceptance.

BREATH MECHANICS

The structure and efficiency of breathing. Free diaphragmatic motion signals safety; shallow, upper-chest breathing often reflects vigilance. Breath frequently changes before pain does, making it an early indicator of system load.
See also: Diaphragm Bracing.

BOX BREATHING

A rhythmic breathing pattern—equal inhale, hold, exhale, hold—used to introduce cadence and perceived safety to an overloaded system. It is a regulation tool rather than a performance technique.
See also: 4-7-8 Breath.

CCJ (CRANIO-CERVICAL JUNCTION)

The anatomical and neurological interface between the skull and the upper cervical spine (occiput–C1–C2). A dense sensorimotor integration zone informing balance, vision, airway behavior, and postural tone. Distortion here can generate widespread, non-local symptoms.
See also: Atlas, Cervical Syndrome Test.

CERVICAL SYNDROME TEST

A clinical assessment evaluating whether head position influences pelvic alignment, leg-length presentation, and global neuromuscular tone. A positive response suggests the upper cervical region is contributing significant load to the system.

COMPENSATION

The body's protective strategy when healthy adaptation is insufficient. Compensation preserves survival and function but is energetically costly. Sustained compensation distorts alignment and eventually produces symptoms. Most chronic pain reflects compensation rather than tissue failure.

CORRECTIVE PHASE

The first phase of the Teeth-to-Toes Roadmap, focused on identifying and reducing the Primary Driver—the distortion currently placing the greatest load on the nervous system. The corrective phase is assessment-driven and interdisciplinary when necessary.
See also: Primary Driver, Sequence.

DAKIN EFFECT

A clinical observation that the same exercise or input can produce opposite outcomes depending on system state, timing, or side. It underscores that exercise is not inherently beneficial; its effect depends on capacity, compensation, and sequence.
See also: Adaptation, Compensation, Sequence.

DIAPHRAGM BRACING

A defensive pattern in which the diaphragm stiffens rather than moves freely. This restricts breathing efficiency, elevates autonomic load, and frequently accompanies pelvic distortion or airway strain.

FUNCTIONAL LEG-LENGTH DIFFERENCE

An apparent difference in leg length caused by pelvic torsion, neuromuscular imbalance, or upper cervical distortion rather than true bone asymmetry. It is state-dependent and may change immediately when the Primary Driver is reduced. Its presence signals unresolved compensation.
See also: Pelvic Torsion, Compensation, Primary Driver.

HYPERVIGILANCE

A nervous-system state in which threat detection overrides rest and clarity. It may present as persistent muscle tension, jaw clenching, shallow breathing, sleep disturbance, or difficulty stabilizing corrections—often without conscious anxiety.

LOAD

The total mechanical, emotional, environmental, and neurological demand placed on the system at a given time. Load determines how quickly capacity is consumed and when compensation becomes necessary.

MAINTENANCE PHASE

The final phase of the Roadmap, focused on preserving alignment, capacity, and adaptability through minimal, intelligent routines and periodic reassessment. Maintenance represents stewardship rather than fragility.

MICRON

One-thousandth of a millimeter. In dentistry and occlusal work, it illustrates that extremely small structural differences can carry meaningful neurological consequences when system tolerance is low.

NEUROLOGICAL ACCEPTANCE

The moment the nervous system recognizes that a meaningful reduction in load has occurred. Often experienced as a spontaneous breath, release, or sense of internal clarity. Acceptance—not force—allows reorganization to consolidate.

PRIMARY DRIVER

The distortion currently placing the greatest organizing demand on the nervous system. Unlike the historical term "primary lesion," the Primary Driver need not involve tissue damage. It refers to the dominant load-producing factor at a specific time. Primary is contextual and may shift as corrections stabilize. Identifying and reducing the Primary Driver determines sequence.

PROPRIOCEPTIVE CHAOS

A disruption in the body's internal sense of position and movement. It may present as imbalance, clumsiness, dizziness, or a persistent feeling of being "off-center." Restoring alignment improves signal clarity.

REFLEXIVE STABILITY

Effortless, automatic organization allowing upright posture without conscious bracing. Lost under overload; restored when primary sources of compensation are reduced.

SEQUENCE

The order in which interventions must occur for corrections to hold. Sequence is discovered through assessment and response, not imposed by theory. Respecting sequence is central to durable recovery.

STABILIZATION PHASE

The second Roadmap phase, focused on teaching the body to maintain improved alignment through tolerable corrective exercise, breath regulation, and pacing. The aim is efficiency and trust—not brute strength.

SYMPATHETIC DOMINANCE

A physiological state marked by elevated muscle tone, shallow breathing, heightened vigilance, and reduced recovery. Common in chronic, load-sensitive systems.

TMJ (TEMPOROMANDIBULAR JOINT)

The joint connecting the jaw to the skull. Neurologically rich and sensitive to occlusal clarity. When the bite becomes unstable, the TMJ often shifts from sensory monitor to stabilizer, increasing cranial and cervical strain.

TONGUE POSTURE

The resting position of the tongue. Influences airway size, facial development, and bite stability. Proper tongue posture supports nasal breathing and reduces compensatory load.

UPPER CERVICAL CARE (NUCCA AND RELATED METHODS)

Precision-based, low-force approaches focused on restoring orientation at the cranio-cervical junction rather than increasing mobility. When applied at the appropriate point in sequence, these methods may produce global effects by restoring sensory clarity at a primary orientation hub.

VILLAGE SQUAT

A foundational human movement and corrective reference pattern used to assess and improve alignment, mobility, and symmetry from the ground up. Though not a formal diagnostic test, it often reveals compensation patterns in major weightbearing joints and the spine.

Bibliography

FOUNDATIONAL NEUROPHYSIOLOGY & SYSTEMS ORGANIZATION (How the nervous system integrates posture, movement, and threat)

Bernstein, Nikolai A. *The Co-ordination and Regulation of Movements.* Oxford: Pergamon Press, 1967.

Guyton, Arthur C., and John E. Hall. *Textbook of Medical Physiology.* 13th ed. Philadelphia: Elsevier, 2015.

Kandel, Eric R., James H. Schwartz, Thomas M. Jessell, Steven A. Siegelbaum, and A. J. Hudspeth. *Principles of Neural Science.* 5th ed. New York: McGraw-Hill, 2012.

Latash, Mark L. *Neurophysiological Basis of Movement.* 2nd ed. Champaign, IL: Human Kinetics, 2008.

Sherrington, Charles S. *The Integrative Action of the Nervous System.* New Haven, CT: Yale University Press, 1906.

MOTOR CONTROL, STABILITY & PROTECTIVE STRATEGIES (Adaptation, compensation, and stiffness as survival logic)

Aruin, Alexander S. 2011. "Enhancing Anticipatory Postural Adjustments: A Novel Approach to Balance Rehabilitation." *Journal of Neurologic Physical Therapy* 35 (1): 5–9.

Dankaerts, Wim, et al. 2006. "Differences in Sitting Postures Are Associated with Non-Specific Chronic Low Back Pain Disorders." *Spine* 31 (6): 698–704.

Hodges, Paul W., and Carolyn A. Richardson. 1996. "Inefficient Muscular Stabilisation of the Lumbar Spine Associated with Low Back Pain." *Spine* 21 (22): 2640–2650.

Hodges, Paul W., and Carolyn A. Richardson. 1999. "Altered Trunk Muscle Recruitment in People with Chronic Low Back Pain with Upper Limb Movements." *Spine* 24 (23): 2643–2651.

Jones, S., et al. 2011. "Individuals with Non-Specific Low Back Pain Use a Trunk Stiffening Strategy to Maintain Upright Posture." *Journal of Electromyography and Kinesiology* 22: 13–20.

McGill, Stuart. *Low Back Disorders: Evidence-Based Prevention and Rehabilitation*. 3rd ed. Champaign, IL: Human Kinetics, 2016.

O'Sullivan, P., et al. 2002. "Posture and Low Back Pain." *Spine* 27: 1238–1244.

PELVIC ASYMMETRY, LOAD TRANSFER & GLOBAL DISTORTION (The mechanical hub of the system)

Lee, Diane, and Linda-Joy Lee. 2014. "Is Pelvic Asymmetry a Cause or a Consequence of Dysfunction?" *Journal of Manual & Manipulative Therapy* 22 (1): 2–12.

Lopes, E., et al. 2006. "Assessment of Muscle Shortening and Static Posture in Children with Persistent Asthma." *European Journal of Pediatrics* 166 (7): 715–721.

Schamberger, Wolfgang. *The Malalignment Syndrome: Implications for Medicine and Sport*. Edinburgh: Churchill Livingstone, 2002.

Schamberger, Wolfgang. *Read My Hips: How to Resolve the 'Hidden Culprit' of Persistent Pain*. Vancouver: Body Align Publishing, 2012.

CRANIO-CERVICAL JUNCTION, PROPRIOCEPTION & ORIENTATION (The compass of the system)

Bolton, Paul S. 2002. "Influence of the Cervical Spine on the Autonomic Nervous System." *Journal of Manipulative and Physiological Therapeutics* 25 (2): S80–S86.

Brandt, Thomas, and Marianne Dieterich. 1994. "Vestibular Syndromes in the Roll Plane." *Annals of Neurology* 36 (3): 337–347.

Brandt, Thomas, and Adolfo M. Bronstein. 2001. "Cervical Vertigo." *Journal of Neurology, Neurosurgery & Psychiatry* 71 (1): 8–12.

Cheung, C., et al. 2010. "The Correlation Between Craniovertebral Angle, Backpack Weights, and Disability Due to Neck Pain in Adolescents." *Journal of Back and Musculoskeletal Rehabilitation* 23: 129–136.

Pettorossi, V., and M. Schieppati. 2014. "Neck Proprioception Shapes Body Orientation and Perception of Motion." *Frontiers in Human Neuroscience* 8: 895.

Richmond, F. J. R., and V. C. Abrahams. 1979. "What Are the Proprioceptors of the Neck?" *Progress in Brain Research* 50: 245–254.

Sutherland, William G. *The Cranial Bowl*. Portland, OR: Osteopathic Publishing Company, 1939.

Treleaven, Julia. 2008. "Sensorimotor Disturbances in Neck Disorders Affecting Postural Stability, Head and Eye Movement Control." *Manual Therapy* 13 (1): 2–11.

JAW, AIRWAY & CRANIOFACIAL INTEGRATION (Bite as sensor, not driver)

Goldstein, L., and H. Makofsky. 2005. "TMD/Facial Pain and Forward Head Posture." *Practical Pain Management* 5 (5): 36–39.

Panagopoulos, John, et al. 2012. "The Relationship Between Cervical Spine Dysfunction and Temporomandibular Disorders." *Journal of Oral Rehabilitation* 39 (9): 628–638.

Solow, Bjørn, and P. Tallgren. 1976. "Head Posture and Craniofacial Morphology." *American Journal of Physical Anthropology* 44 (3): 417–435.

Visscher, Cornelis M., et al. 2020. "The Clinical Aspects of Temporomandibular Disorders and Cervical Spine Dysfunction." *Journal of Oral Rehabilitation* 47 (4): 380–402.

AUTONOMIC LOAD, AFFECT & PREDICTIVE PROCESSING (Threat, capacity, and state-dependent physiology)

Clark, Andy. *Surfing Uncertainty: Prediction, Action, and the Embodied Mind*. Oxford: Oxford University Press, 2016.

Friston, Karl. 2010. "The Free-Energy Principle: A Unified Brain Theory?" *Nature Reviews Neuroscience* 11: 127–138.

Moseley, G. Lorimer, and David Butler. *Explain Pain Supercharged*. Adelaide: NOI Group Publications, 2017.

Seth, Anil. *Being You: A New Science of Consciousness*. London: Faber & Faber, 2021.

Apkarian, A., et al. 2004. "Chronic Back Pain Is Associated with Decreased Prefrontal and Thalamic Gray Matter Density." *Journal of Neuroscience* 24 (46).

Deuchars, J., and I. Edwards. 2007. "Bad Posture Could Raise Your Blood Pressure." *Journal of Neuroscience* 27 (24).

Henderson, Fraser C. Sr., et al. 2017. "Neurological and Spinal Manifestations of the Ehlers–Danlos Syndromes." *American Journal of Medical Genetics Part C* 175 (1): 195–211.

Rosario, J., et al. 2014. "Differences and Similarities in Postural Alterations Caused by Sadness and Depression." *Journal of Bodywork and Movement Therapies* 18 (4): 540–544.

MANUAL THERAPY & INTEGRATION MODELS (Hands-on traditions informing modern sequencing)

Biedermann, Hans. *Manual Therapy in Children*. Edinburgh: Churchill Livingstone, 1990.

Rolf, Ida P. *Rolfing: Structural Integration*. Rochester, VT: Healing Arts Press, 1977.

St. John, Paul. *Neuromuscular Therapy Manual*. Ocala, FL: St. John Seminars Press, 1990.

NEUROMUSCULAR RE-EDUCATION & REHAB FRAMEWORKS

Hanna, Thomas. *Somatics: Reawakening the Mind's Control of Movement, Flexibility, and Health*. New York: Da Capo Press, 1988.

Janda, Vladimir. *Muscle Function Testing*. London: Butterworths, 1983.

Kendall, Florence Peterson, Elizabeth Kendall McCreary, and Patricia Geise Provance. *Muscles: Testing and Function*. 4th ed. Baltimore: Williams & Wilkins, 1993.

Kolar, Pavel, et al. *Clinical Rehabilitation*. Prague: Rehabilitation Prague School Press, 2009.

APPLIED CLINICAL SYNTHESIS & CONTEMPORARY SOURCES (Living models and interdisciplinary integration)

Dakin, Geoff. *The Body Mechanic's Handbook*. 2nd ed. Calgary: Vitruvian Publishing, 2018.

Nestor, James. *Breath: The New Science of a Lost Art*. New York: Riverhead Books, 2020.

Dakin, G., Westersund, C., & Scholten, J. 2025. "Teeth-to-Toes: Evolving the Way We Treat Pain and Dysfunction." Live interdisciplinary lecture delivered at the Hyo Maier Centre for Dental Excellence, Calgary, Alberta, October 8, 2025.

Vásquez, Javier. 2025. "The Modern Oral Physician." Live lecture delivered at the Hyo Maier Centre for Dental Excellence, Calgary, Alberta, December 5, 2025.

Acknowledgments

No book is ever written in isolation. This one—perhaps more than most—is a chorus rather than a solo. It carries the fingerprints, questions, disagreements, refinements, and generosity of an entire clinical lineage.

Although I am listed as the primary author, and although Dr. Curtis Westersund and Dr. Jeff Scholten stand here as collaborators and co-architects of this work, the deeper truth is simple: nothing in these pages was built alone. The Teeth-to-Toes model is not the product of a single mind. It is what happens when three disciplines choose to think together, test together, disagree respectfully, and follow physiology wherever it leads—even when it leads beyond the borders of our original training.

Long before the three of us found a shared language, there were teachers whose influence shaped the way I see the human body. Three in particular left marks deep enough that their fingerprints can still be found throughout these chapters.

To Geoff Gluckman,
You were the first to show me that movement could be both corrective and diagnostic—that posture was not a static image to critique, but a living dialogue between the body and gravity. You challenged early assumptions and replaced them with a way of seeing that felt radical at the time and obvious in hindsight.

Long before I had the language to describe what I was witnessing in clinic, I had your lens. The Alignment First Protocol grew from seeds planted during those early years of study with you. For your generosity, your mentorship, and your belief in my work long before it had a name, I remain profoundly grateful.

To Dr. Wolfgang Schamberger,

Your books—*The Malalignment Syndrome* and *Read My Hips*—gave an entire generation of clinicians permission to trust what our eyes and hands were already detecting. You legitimized what many of us sensed but could not yet articulate.

In 1989, you told my graduating class that it takes thirty years to truly understand the human body. I remember the silence in the room. For some, it felt discouraging. For me, it became a compass—an invitation into apprenticeship rather than ambition.

Three decades later, when you reached out asking about my research and exploring the relationship between bite and posture—speaking to me as a colleague rather than a former student—it became one of the great honors of my career. Your curiosity, rigor, and humility continue to shape my thinking. This book carries your influence with deep respect.

To Paul St. John,

Your pioneering work in Neuromuscular Therapy reframed how I understood the body's interconnected systems. You taught me that patterns are not merely distortions to be corrected—they are messages. They are the nervous system's attempt to remain organized under overwhelming load.

Much of the nuance in these pages—the blending of biomechanics with neurophysiology and lived experience—rests on foundations you laid decades ago. Your willingness to follow complexity without oversimplifying it gave me permission to build a model capable of holding the body's full story.

These three teachers offered lenses, frameworks, and challenges at pivotal moments. Without their influence, the Alignment First Protocol would not exist. Neither would the Teeth-to-Toes model. Neither would this book.

I am equally grateful to the many colleagues and friends who read early drafts, asked uncomfortable questions, challenged assumptions, and sharpened ideas. Thoughtful critique is an act of generosity. This book is stronger because it was questioned.

In particular, I want to thank Dr. Jeff Scholten, Dr. Curtis Westersund, and Dr. Christian Leonhardt for their intellectual rigor, candor, and willingness to engage deeply with ideas that refuse to stay neatly inside one discipline. Collaboration of that kind is rare. It is also essential.

And finally, to the patients.

Every refinement in this book was earned in a room with a real person whose nervous system was trying to solve a problem. They trusted us with their stories, their persistence, and their hope. The body remains the only true author here. We are merely the scribes.

To every nervous system fighting to be seen, and to every practitioner trying to see it clearly: may this book serve as a bridge. May it help you reduce load, restore coherence, and rediscover capacity.

And may we never stop listening.

www.ingramcontent.com/pod-product-compliance
Lightning Source LLC
LaVergne TN
LVHW010727061126
851857LV00014B/1370
* 9 7 8 0 9 9 5 1 8 2 6 7 7 *